A Full House—But Empty

A Full House—But Empty

Angus Munro

iUniverse, Inc.
New York Lincoln Shanghai

A Full House—But Empty

iUniverse books may be ordered through booksellers or by contacting:

iUniverse
2021 Pine Lake Road, Suite 100
Lincoln, NE 68512
www.iuniverse.com
1-800-Authors (1-800-288-4677)

ISBN: 978-0-595-43719-1 (pbk)
ISBN: 978-0-595-88050-8 (ebk)

Printed in the United States of America

Acknowledgements

Many thanks to the following persons for their unstinting encouragement and constructive prodding in keeping me focused on this project.

Kudos to my endearing family for getting me started.

Thankfully, to my dear, Linda Howard, for her collaboration on the title of my book.

Gratefully, to William Greenleaf for his valuable literary input and tenacious support.

Appreciatively, to Kristin Oomen of iUniverse. Inc., for her ongoing support, and to Jan Howarth, editorial consultant to iUniverse, Inc., for her literary expertise.

Preface

Every book is intended to convey a message. I am certain that one would be somewhat puzzled regarding the title of my book, *A Full House—But Empty*. My father, not by choice but by circumstance, became a single parent. I believe he inherently possessed a bachelor's mentality—not in terms of womanizing, but in other pursuits, such as playing poker. Thus the term, *A Full House* the other half of my title—*But Empty*—actually refers to my ongoing insular existence living in the shadow of a house that seemed like a mini Grand Central Station.

At age eleven, I found myself burdened with heavy family responsibilities when I became partially responsible for minding my younger sister and having to maintain our living quarters in terms of cleaning, marketing, and preparing our meals. Along with those duties, I cleaned up after poker games, parties, and people who simply popped in on a daily basis to shoot the breeze with my father. We were constantly faced with people from out of town coming to stay with us for a visit and/or to get reestablished in Vancouver or elsewhere. It seems to me that my father must have been repulsed by the thought of ever being alone.

Because of this chaotic and unorthodox lifestyle, I had no heroes. Even among our large circle of friends, relatives, and acquaintances I couldn't find anyone to emulate or to go to for help with my basic growing-up needs, concerns, and frustrations. Even in this chaotic circle, I still had the most wonderful father in the universe.

In our kitchen, at the head of the table, there sat a large straw armchair reserved exclusively for my father. One of my father's poker pals stopped by one evening. As my father was out, I was sitting in his chair. The poker pal said, "What the hell are you doing sitting in your father's chair?" He was not being facetious—he actually reprimanded me by citing my unworthiness to be seated at the head of the table. I must have temporarily forgotten that I was a domestic servant before I was a son!

Strangely enough, living in that environment actually gave me a certain amount of humility that I found very beneficial in my later years. To begin with, I have been blessed with boundless energy, and, along with that, I am a consummate neat freak. My boyhood home, regardless of the commotion from parties and poker games, was maintained immaculately by this unappreciated skinny and somewhat neurotic little kid.

Because of the circumstances, I lived in a totally adult world. I was so distraught and confused that one traumatic event involving a stolen pen was enough to push me over the edge and caused me to drop out of school at the age of fourteen. I was a loner living an insular life that seemed to be without purpose or structure.

I am no celebrity. I am no self-help success story, never having been plagued with drugs or alcohol, abusive behavior, or crime. Eventually I picked up the pieces of my life and forged ahead. In hindsight, I believe I had a strong desire to be successful and to achieve challenging goals. I also had a longing to be recognized and needed for my productivity. At home, however, I seemed to be burdened with roadblocks and displacement, and I was constantly subjected to the inundation of unwelcome guests.

An interested colleague once casually asked me if I had had a planned and structured background or if I simply had played with the deck dealt to me. That person had no knowledge of my background—and knew nothing about our poker games. Without further elaboration, I stated that I'd simply played with the deck dealt to me. I quietly and shockingly thought, *What a profoundly worded statement to direct to me.*

I vividly recall my third-grade teacher attempting to instill the following simple message to her very young students:

> If a task once begun,
> Never leave it till it's done,
> Be it ever great or small,
> Do it well or not at all!

My father had simply said, "Do the right thing." My own motto throughout my life, in the work scene and privately, has always been, "Whatever you do, follow through."

Ironically, my mentor and greatest teacher (often through osmosis) was my father. Apart from his social activities, he was, for many years, an outside foreman for a large oil and coal company. He never ever missed a day at work. He always kept me informed on employee-related issues and how he addressed them, and we discussed the decision-making process. He was very strong in terms of labor relations; however, in the process, he was loyal and supportive to the general manager of the company. He saw the entire picture and he would explain in detail how one must, through sagacious balancing, bring everything together to benefit both sides. Both the outside men and the office staff attended the parties at our house. They all loved and admired my father for his great attributes and contributions in terms of fairness and compassion and unstinting dedication to the organization. He accepted all challenges at work with alacrity, and explained to me the importance of accepting responsibilities thrust upon one. These conversations were great quiet moments.

The humility I learned as a youngster benefited me in later life. On numerous occasions when I had a staffing complement of fifty-five to seventy employees, I would often clean the office myself over the weekend. The cleaning was necessary because of certain untidy employees and inadequate janitorial services. We neat freaks have no boundaries, and modesty prevails—we simply seek the end result knowing it is often viewed unappreciatively.

My father had a decorous mother. Thus, we learned by emulation proper table manners from our father—a great social reassurance. We knew to stand when guests entered our home and to be certain they received the available seating accommodations. On public transportation we were instructed to give up our seats to all women, older men, and any person with an infirmity.

During our early youth, my younger sister mentioned that a good friend to our older sister was working as a cashier at a theater located in a skid row part of downtown Vancouver. That brought forth our joint negative smirks and comments. Watching us and hearing our comments, my father was absolutely outraged and immediately took over the conversation, succinctly inquiring, "And what duties would that young lady perform differently at an upscale movie theater?" He had us on that one. And he spent several minutes telling us never to make defamatory comments about anyone who is doing an honest day's work. We got his message clearly and profoundly.

Because I was a Depression-born child, I always believed that to have a job is a privilege, and it is my duty to fulfill what is expected of me. However, it has always been important to me to be able to work well with others and to inject humor in fulfilling my specific duties. A friendly and harmonious atmosphere in the workplace is important. In the process, there is a definite need for balance between responsibility and fun. I recall an incident when one of my young tennis protégés, whose parents owned a delicatessen, helped me deliver an order of food for one of our office potluck luncheons. I had a staff of about fifty-five people and I suggested that my young friend stay for lunch and mingle with our group. He was very outgoing and enjoyed the experience of seeing me off the tennis courts in a different role.

Some weeks later he informed me that he needed my assistance in resolving an employee problem. He was attending college but was responsible for working in the family deli some evenings after school and weekends. There was a young lady also working at the deli that initially worked well with him and also enjoyed having fun and sharing humor with him. He said, however, that after a few weeks, the humor overtook her work duties and her job just became fun and games to her. I responded, "Getting the work done is your primary consideration. All else is secondary." He agreed: no balance, no job.

As a school dropout, I received most of my education, by necessity and empirically, through my work experience. When my ex-wife and I arrived in California, many newcomers were seeking job opportunities through employment agencies. Shortly after our arrival in Los Angeles, I accompanied my wife to one of the employment agencies where she had an appointment to leave an application. After her interview, the employment specialist inquired if the young man in the waiting room was her husband. She said, "Yes." He made some laudatory comments regarding my appearance and stated he would like to interview me also for a position. Needless to say, I was happy to meet with him and I explained that I had a work plan in place.

Two employment specialists shared the same office. There was a young man just completing an interview with the other specialist and, after saying farewell to the other applicant, he joined our conversation. Both specialists looked at me and laughingly explained that the applicant grammatically murdered the English language and could never successfully go beyond an initial interview. I politely smiled but made no comment. What they unfortunately did not realize was that, when they sent him on interviews, his performance reflected jointly on their poor judgment as well as his poor grammar. They should have leveled with him and sent him to a language specialist for help. The end result could have been a winning situation for both instead of ongoing, unproductive rejection for both.

When I was a new director of business services at the largest hospital in Alaska, I was overwhelmed with the amount of work necessary to bring my areas of responsibility to an acceptable standard. Upon my arrival to work, I would frequently see one of the radiologists, who was responsible for a high-volume outpatient services department, beating a trail to one of the assistant administrator's office to complain about internal systems. I recall that the assistant administrator was under forty years old (friendly but slightly arrogant) and the wall behind his desk was lined with impressive degrees and certificates. Needless to say, I saw those as more proverbial nails to add to this grade-school dropout's coffin. Unfortunately, the radiologist was discontented with administration and freely expressed his views regarding their incompetence to me. He was very affable and extremely engaging when espousing his discontent. Finally, I asked one of my key persons in our outpatient admitting office for input regarding the radiologist's discontent. His comprehensive explanation enabled me to bring forth the true source and identification of the problem, and I was able to resolve it. The radiologist was elated; however, the wall behind my desk still remained blank.

While I was working at one hospital during my career, I stopped by my office on a Sunday morning to pick-up some prepared material I required for a meeting at a sister hospital in another city the following day. I was planning to leave for the meeting after I picked up my material. I stopped by our admitting office to say hello, and the admitting representative informed me that she had just sent a patient home. The patient was to have an elective surgery (non-emergency), but her physician was listed on our medical records delinquency list. In layman's terms, physicians who were behind in completing their medical record patient charts were penalized—by not being allowed to admit their non-emergency cases. In all fairness, it was a very frustrating situation when patient charts were not completed in a timely fashion for numerous reasons. However, the admitting representative informed me that the patient had arranged to take two weeks off from work to have the surgery. Additionally, she had driven several miles to come to the hospital and she had received no advance warning regarding this situation. She was shocked that she was being sent home because of a situation she did not understand.

I immediately contacted the physician and informed him that I was approving the admission and that he needed to address his problem with medical records the following day. He thanked me profusely and I had the admitting representative call the patient and have her return to the hospital immediately. I waited until the patient returned to the hospital before starting my trip.

Awaiting my return to the office on Tuesday was a very caustic letter from my admitting manager, who happened to be a nun. She was overly protective of her staff and informed me that I had interfered inappropriately in the above situation. I rationally blamed her shortsightedness on immaturity and stated that my concern related to the patient with no reflection on our admitting staff. In these situations, I always recalled my father saying, "Do the right thing regardless of the situation and outcome!" Years later after leaving her religious order that admitting manager sent me a letter seeking employment. I was working at another hospital, and, after reading her letter, I found my wastebasket staring me in the face!

Closing thoughts:

What do these stories really convey—other than appearing to be a potpourri of separate tales? They each reflect by example how I personally view incidents in my life in terms of responsibility, recognition, personal conduct, and considering the needs of others.

- Yes, as a child I lived in a mishmash and hectic environment and somehow I had to put it all together and accept adult responsibilities.

- And the reward for my efforts should not have been some idiot superficially telling me about sitting in my father's chair. It should have been recognition and appreciation.

- I did the clean-up work at home as an accepted job assignment. I didn't make the rules; however, in order to survive, I had to abide by them.

- I dropped out of school based on circumstances and immaturity.

- I had a clean slate—no drugs, alcohol, or abusive behavior.

- I ran with my father's better qualities. I had an innate sense of distinction.

- As a director, I wasn't above participating in grunt work; I valued teamwork.

- Demonstrating proper personal manners in all settings is complimentary to yourself and those in your presence. Dignity should always prevail.

- I have to agree with the infamous Nikita Khrushchev: "It is not the work that is dirty, but rather the conscience." There is glory in fulfilling the task, not demeaning it.

- I believe in a balance of both harmony and productivity in the workplace.

- If an applicant has a poor grasp of his language, tell him, help him, and don't embarrass him.

- Accepting responsibility and successfully resolving issues cannot be displayed as a plaque or degree on your office wall. It is an obligation to fulfill these tasks proficiently and with alacrity.

- Do the right thing regardless of the situation or outcome. Dignity and respect for others should be the hallmark. And include yourself in the process.

Introduction

After celebrating my thirty-ninth year in hospital administration, and reaching the age of seventy-two, I decided, in 2003, to retire. This was an important decision for me, having always been labeled a workaholic possessed with somewhat boundless, nervous energy. The work regimentation had been so ingrained in me, at such an early age, I could hardly comprehend how I would "pick-up the pieces" and move on.

I once married the woman of my dreams, whom I love to this day, but never liked. We have been divorced for years, and, after a very brief second marriage, I have been single most of my life, which has given me plenty of time to live my life as a practicing workaholic and an ardent tennis bum—both being separate ends of the spectrum and often having negative connotations.

After two weeks of retirement, I was called upon to spend a few days taking care of my two great nephews. Grant is eight and Kyle is almost eleven and they were out of school for the summer. No shyness exists in my relationship with my nephews. They plan our movies and social events and other activities. I am simply the third kid—I just have gray hair and I pick-up the tab. I unequivocally do not comprehend their computer games and other related applications and paraphernalia. Conversely, it would be difficult for them to comprehend the simplicity of my childhood, when I lived in a world of limited media—only radio, newspapers, magazines, and mainly adult movies. (And no fast food restaurants!)

Frankly, I was just about my nephews' age when I spent the happiest years of my life—between the ages of seven and eleven years old. I was residing in the most beautiful city in the world—Vancouver, British Columbia. That particular time period, from 1938 to 1942, saw the end of the Depression and the beginning of World War II. I did have to review my family roots when I wrote about that period of my life, but all of the memories relating to my precious day-to-day life during that period in my life are very close and clear in my mind.

My great nephews' father Paul is married to my niece Robin. While having breakfast with Paul and Kyle one morning, I was discussing my childhood years and reminiscing by telling anecdotes and short stories. Paul is very interested in family history, and he suggested that I start jotting some of my experiences down on paper. During the conversation, I mentioned that I would like to write a Waltonesque story about my childhood that our lads might find interesting to read.

I wrote about my childhood, covering a four-year period. When my story was finished and I had presented it to my family, Robin, Paul, and I sat down to discuss what they had just read.

Paul said, "Uncle Gus, you're just getting started—you should continue your story."

"Paul, do you mean I should write a full autobiography?"

"Yes! You've shared so many of your experiences with us—we know you have the ingredients for an interesting book. Also, you know how keen I am on our family history. It's important to all of us. And you play a key role, being a senior member of our family."

While pondering over his comments, I did submit my childhood story to a newspaper as a special feature, and it was immediately accepted. When Paul heard about this, he ebulliently commented, "Uncle Gus, that's a great compliment to your writing skills, but I still urge you to hold off printing that article. You should continue your writing!"

"Okay, Paul, I'll take your advice. Let's see what happens."

The Munro family came from Ross-shire, Scotland, in 1830 and settled in southern Ontario, Canada. The family today represents about nine generations, who still reside on the same beautiful and bountiful farmland complete with lakes and woodlands. Around 1905, my entrepreneurial grandfather left his Ontario property in trust with the Munro clan and took his family via covered wagon to newly opened settler lands in Saskatchewan to become a wheat farmer. My father, at age five, was the oldest child, and he remembered that long journey. My grandfather settled in southern Saskatchewan, and during the course of his life he acquired seven sections of land and was considered the most prosperous and well-respected farmer in the community.

When my father married, my grandfather leased other farmland for him to work so he could establish himself as an individual. After my father received funds from his first wheat crop—a sizeable amount for those days—he attended a wild poker game at the local grain elevator. In the prairie towns, the grain elevator seemed to be the leading gathering place for male social activity. By the time my father left the poker game and returned home, he had but one can of strawberry jam to present to my mother. One could only imagine the anguish and related thoughts of both the giver and receiver regarding that can of strawberry preserves.

My father decided that farming was not for him, and he moved to Vancouver. Although my father worked long, hard hours farming, my grandfather was not too enchanted with him because of the poker incident and, presumably, other related issues. Unfortunately, my grandfather died shortly thereafter, leaving everything to his second son. My father was devastated at being excluded from his father's will. The Depression had started and my father was a farm boy, occupationally untrained for city life. It was difficult for him to find work to support his family.

As the Depression continued to deepen, my father journeyed back to Saskatchewan in 1934 to see his brother as a last appeal for help. He received nothing. He returned to Vancouver unexpectedly one evening. His return took my mother—and a male companion—by surprise. The companion jumped out of the nearest window and ran for cover.

I was unaware of whatever confrontation transpired between my father and mother that evening, as I heard no commotion. However, I simultaneously became very seriously ill. At that time, my sister Marjorie was still an infant, I was three years old, and my sister Laura was six years old.

1

At the age of three, I suffered from appendicitis and spent seven weeks in the Vancouver General Hospital. Little did I know or understand at the time that my mother and father were seriously struggling with their relationship, and that the future of our family life was hanging in the balance.

Upon my arrival home from the hospital, I was immediately put into my bed, which was a large crib that had been placed in the living room. As soon as I settled in, I asked my six-year-old sister Laura, "Where is mummy?"

"She doesn't live here anymore," she stated flatly.

Her words shocked me. I started thrashing around and screaming hysterically, "Mummy, Mummy!" My father rushed into the room to rescue me and to pacify me.

"It's okay. Everything is going to be okay. We're here with you now." I continued to cry hysterically. I felt dejected. Why did I seem to be the only one upset with this tragic news? I did not comprehend that my mother had been gone from home for seven weeks. This was old news to Laura, but fresh news to me.

Fortunately, to cover my mother's departure from our home, we were blessed with two wonderful housekeepers who tried to pick-up the pieces. They had been provided at no cost to us by the Provincial Social Services. One or the other came daily during the week to take care of our needs. They were so kind and motherly that being with them helped our days to flow freely. My father said on many occasions that they spent more time playing and taking care of us individually than they did fulfilling household chores. He frankly preferred it that way. He said he would return home daily to three happy smiling faces and a somewhat disheveled apartment. Dishevelment was of no importance to him.

One day, my sister Laura and I looked in the window of a bakeshop that was located half a block from our apartment. In the center of the display window was a beautiful white cake with a maraschino cherry right in the middle on top. I was five and knew nothing about the Depression and how poor we were. When we returned home, I told my father about the beautiful cake and wondered if he could buy it for us.

He asked, "Are you certain you want that cake?"

I replied, "More than anything else."

Apparently, it was uncommon for me to ask for anything. I recall my father reaching into his pocket and pulling out what little money he had. He started counting his change on the kitchen table to see if he had enough to purchase the cake.

Again, he reiterated to me, "Are you certain you really want that cake?"

"Yes!"

He gave my sister the money to purchase it for us. I thought that cake was the nicest gesture he ever bestowed on me. Even as a little kid, I was very moved to see him count what little money he had to buy that cake for me. I didn't know it at the time, but I am certain now that he needed that money for food for himself for the following day.

There was a wonderful French Canadian family who lived about two blocks from our apartment. They were a large family, and their children were reaching adulthood. The boys brought their girlfriends and the girls their boyfriends, and they gathered around our large kitchen table with my father and others and played poker. (They used The Eddy Match Company's staple wooden matches presumably when not flush—in place of money.) I particularly loved their mother, a very small frail lady with a very thick French Canadian accent. I also admired her beautiful daughter, Rosie. The girls and guys would stop by and take Laura and me to the neighborhood movies with them. Sometimes, when my father went out in the evening, Rosie or other family members came to take care of us, and we loved it. They were our family, too. The mother welcomed us to their home at any time, spoiling us with goodies.

During that period, our apartment always seemed full of people. A barber-friend of my father came one day and gave me a haircut. When he was finished, he handed me a mirror and I screamed bloody murder. It looked very bad to me. My father and the barber laughed hysterically at my reaction. I hid under the kitchen table refusing to budge and remained there until the barber left. They both thought it was funny. I must have stayed under that table for quite a while; I was so angry at receiving what I thought to be a rotten haircut—my first and last haircut from him, poor guy.

Laura took me to school on my first day, as she attended the same school. I was the only child in the classroom that first day without a parent present. I silently addressed my feeling of aloneness by believing the other students were babies who needed their mothers to bring them to class. Laura was very popular and she was actively involved in school concerts with her tap dancing skills. She was so beautiful and always looked so nice. I was very proud that she was my sister. She tried to take good care of her little brother—attempting to be a surrogate mother. I was very dependent on her in many ways. I loved her very much.

When I was seven, we moved in with another family who were faced with similar financial circumstances. The father was a divorced man who cared for five children, but he was fully employed with a roofing company. My father, during this period, was able to obtain only sporadic employment. Under those conditions, we moved into their rented house to see if we could develop a good rapport by pooling our resources and co-existing harmoniously.

I felt no sense of excitement in moving in with the other family because they were total strangers to me. We were allocated a couple of rooms in their cramped living quarters and we had the feeling that we were simply camping out. I hated living there and was hopeful that this new arrangement would be temporary. I felt no kinship with this family—and little for my own, as a matter of fact, excluding Laura. I quietly kept to myself most of the time during this period.

To me, it was all a very drab existence. My life experiences and observations, sadly at my early age, led me to expect the worst because it seemed the most inevitable. The deprivation of adequate living quarters only compounded my existence of permanently being faced with a single parent.

At age seven, I never even thought about the fact that we were in the midst of a horrible Depression with national suffering everywhere. My personal expectations clearly indicated that nothing but ongoing concessions would be in the offing. I always expected the worst around every corner. I realized from the day I returned home from the hospital at age three that I had control of nothing but hurt and deprivation. And I had no support group—just skinny little me trying to go with the flow. I felt totally alone.

After a few months of living together, the fathers located a larger house and we planned to move at the end of the school year. Aside from sharing similar marital difficulties, both fathers had been farmers from the Canadian wheat provinces. Our combined families represented ten people—our two fathers and eight children: The Inglehart family consisted of the father, Lloyd, Lois (16), Dorothy (14), Gordon (12), Cecil (10), and Rita (7). Our family consisted of our father, Leonard, Laura (10), me (7), and Marjorie (4). Apart from this human group, our household also included two goats and a pen full of chickens—including a couple of roosters to ensure posterity. The goats and chickens belonged to the Inglehart family.

Quite suddenly, because of the anticipated move, I felt a resurgence being uplifted and a unifying bond with the other family. I ebulliently looked forward to our move. With these positive thoughts and anticipation, I immediately bonded with Cecil, who became my favorite family member. We became inseparable.

We were both looking forward to moving to our new home. He and I took the streetcar at the end of our final day of school to the new house and we were excited beyond belief to explore our new surroundings. The house was located on a sloping hill facing False Creek Flats with open meadows facing the front of the property, which would sustain our goats with luscious grass and clover. Surrounding the grasslands were deciduous trees and bushes for our goats to consume. The foliage and space would provide endless areas for us to play in and explore. At long last, I felt "at home," and each day seemed to be filled with excitement beyond my anticipation or imagination. The excitement was overwhelming for both Cecil and me, as we explored the neighborhood and flatlands. We had so much fun hanging out together and laughing at our own corny jokes. We spent our summer holidays outdoors, combing the neighborhood and having a great time.

During the first week in the new house, our family had our meals in the kitchen and the other family had their meals in the dining room. However, at the end of the first week we became one family and sat at newly designated places in the dining room—and the kitchen for breakfast.

Because of family circumstances, Lloyd's daughter Lois had left school after the eighth grade to assume the responsibility of caring for the family and fulfilling household duties. She was wonderful and I soon both loved and respected her. I fulfilled her every request without hesitation. Even at my young age, I realized the huge family responsibilities that she had readily accepted without compromise. On top of that, she had become responsible for three additional children in our family, too. I adored her and I believe the feeling was mutual.

Unlike me, Cecil was not grateful to Lois. He viewed her as having unwarranted dictatorial powers over him and he challenged every one of her requests. I adored them both and removed myself from their frequently quarrelsome relationship. I believe they both appreciated my neutrality. Cecil was the culprit in my unexpressed opinion. Lois simply should have kicked his butt occasionally and sent him flying. She was a noncombatant person, relying on just a war of words with him.

Our inclusion in the Inglehart family added four additional members to their household; however, my father was an excellent cook and he helped inside whenever possible. Everyone loved his ham hocks and beans, homemade pea soup, beef stew, and his not-to-be-forgotten tomato onion cream soup. Dad also continued to cook old Scottish family recipes, too, prepared in one large frying pan. He actively participated in fulfilling all of the outside chores relating to maintenance of our livestock and gardens. My father's active participation in fulfilling a successful unification of our two families did not go unnoticed by me, and I responded by defusing my negative feelings toward him.

One Saturday morning, shortly after our move, I was awakened by the sounds of hammering of nails and a loud conversation taking place the lot adjacent to ours. I quickly dressed and ran outside to see what was happening. Dad and Lloyd and a couple of their friends were building a goat shed and a chicken coop simultaneously. They were surreptitiously usurping the empty lot and even had had the audacity to install a large wire-fenced area where the poultry could meander. They built a small unit to house our pet rabbits as well.

I was shocked at this activity and I wondered if one of our neighbors would report our intrusion and activities to the rightful owner of that vacant lot. I frankly thought I was living with a group of pirates.

I decided to lay low and spend my morning in a safer environment, among our Gravenstein apple trees in the front yard and the two gigantically beautiful lilac bushes that adorned and encircled the front gate entrance. I loved the fragrance of our lilac bushes after a spring rain. We had a small overgrown flower garden patch on one side of the house that I claimed without opposition, and I spent the day there pulling weeds. I was resourceful and sometimes pushy in asking our neighbors for slips from their plants to include in my garden patch. For some unknown reason, they were always willing to comply. Along with the flowers, I had prolific rhubarb plants that produced enough to share with much of the neighborhood in spring.

We cultivated both properties immediately and used them as kitchen gardens. Dad planted and maintained the house garden and Lloyd was responsible for the adjacent lot garden. Our potato crop was our mainstay on both properties; however, we also grew many salad vegetables, peas, green beans, and other vegetables. I must confess, with the inclusion of the adjacent lot and all of the construction, gardening activities, and other embellishments like fencing, our little compound appeared more utilitarian than monolithically unattractive.

Our house, basement, grounds, and sheds were neatly kept and maintained—always free of clutter, junk, or debris. Supplies of fuel products, such as heater and furnace wood, and sawdust for our cooking/hot water kitchen range, were neatly contained in our basement, along with gardening implements. All feed supplies were contained in our chicken pen and goat shed. Our homestead was not an eyesore to the neighborhood.

Gordon, Cecil, and I were never happy when a truckload of firewood arrived. We hated having to haul cords of wood into our basement by wheelbarrow, and pile it all neatly in a designated space. That chore always seemed to occur on a hot summer day. Our fathers critically reviewed our completed chores to be certain we performed them correctly. It was an early lesson in regimentation.

With ten mouths to feed in those Depression years, sustaining an ongoing supply of food was paramount to our existence. We had no refrigerator—only a wooden icebox lined in metal to contain the ice and to keep our perishable foods and liquids fresh. We received new blocks of ice each week. We kids crowded around the iceman's truck, as he would give us small sample pieces to quench our thirst on hot summer days.

My father had an informal agreement (I now assume somewhat nefarious, but he did have a key for the locked gate) to obtain fruit from an orchard in the southern part of Vancouver. There was a bountiful variety of fruit trees in the orchard. In season, we three boys and my father would stand at the rear of the streetcar with gunnysacks or other containers filled with apples, cherries, pears, and plums. We boys were totally embarrassed when other passengers had to squeeze by us and our over-loaded containers. The streetcar conductors must have realized our plight, as they treated us with deference during those awkward trips. People seemed kinder in those difficult Depression days.

To supplement our food supply, we found many vacant properties that yielded loads of wild blackberries, and parasite stumps loaded with huckleberry plants. We also went on neighborhood wild blueberry picking excursions to Lulu Island—children and adults sitting in the back of a neighbor's truck and joyfully singing the latest songs. My father would also make various rounds to the fish canneries and obtain free salmon that was always delicious and fresh. He also received samples of unprocessed sugar from the docks, and we made preserves.

During the season for blueberry picking, two or three adult unmarried daughters of our family friends would come to our house and spend the entire day making delicious pies and other pastries. It was a blessing for us and a godsend for Lois. I especially loved rhubarb pie, and it was fun to have pies from my very own flower-patch crop. If I was low on supply, I could always "surreptitiously" gather some from the neighborhood. Those daughters were so kind to devote time baking for us. Even Cecil was at his grateful best with these ladies, hoping to receive preferential treatment during the distribution period. What a phony, rapacious brat! However, I was a beneficiary of some of his shenanigans, and never ever complained, thus placing myself in the same category. People were so kind and giving of themselves during those Depression years in their efforts to help others. These "cooking visits" were a special, much-appreciated treat. There was an air of excitement whenever one was planned.

With one of these visits imminent, Cecil, during one of his infrequent solemn moods, asked me if I realized that—in his simple terms—we were "borderline poor."

I said, "What are you talking about? We have a great life and a wonderful home."

"Gus, we are a very poor family. There is a serious Depression. So many people are out of work because there are no jobs. Everybody is broke and on relief."

"I still believe we have a great family and a happy life. We go to the movies every week. We have plenty of food on our table. We have gardens, apples, and clothing and shoes."

"Gus you don't understand—we don't have very much money."

"Cecil, your father works every day during the week with the roofing company and the money is probably in his trunk. And my father works when he can!"

"Gus, we are poor, so forget it."

Cecil could be a real brat and he could be very confrontational and stubborn with the other kids in the house. Lois often had to intercede. He would brag to me when he was being confrontational. There were times when I was his only friend in the family and we laughed about it. He was always so agreeable with me and we had happy times. On no occasion did he ever take umbrage when we discussed issues such as our state of finances.

He, too, was a motherless, sensitive soul, and he had had more than his share of disappointment in his young life as well. I realized that I was his favorite person in the whole family. He accepted me at face value and never ever questioned my loyalty—making our relationship free from mistrust or toil. I quietly stood behind, but enjoyed watching him when he was revving up the troops to do verbal battle. He sure could rile them up. Recounting the aftermath, we would roar. On rare occasions, we would have a brief falling out. We would simply give each other the cold shoulder. Shortly thereafter, we would look at each and start laughing and that was it. Our disagreements never lasted more than a couple of hours, if that long.

2

We sold our extra goat's milk to people afflicted with tuberculosis, as it was very beneficial to their condition. And I delivered the milk. On numerous occasions the goats would get loose from pasture and raid the neighborhood flower and vegetable gardens. I was usually home from school before the other lads, and Lois would instruct me to retrieve the goats immediately. The neighbors would scream at me and I would grab the goats and run like hell. As I think about it now, I realize that they were truly benevolent neighbors, as they never ever called the police. Screaming at me seemed enough to soothe their anger.

Some years later, my younger sister Marjorie attended a teenage party, looking like the belle of the ball. One young man, during introductions, pointed to her and shouted,

"I remember you and your family. You had all of those damn goats!"

Two brothers, aged four and five, lived a block away from our house. They were cheeky little brats. They knew every swear word in the book. Cecil and I always wanted to kick their little butts and send them home. However, they adored my father and loved coming to our yard, especially after the baby goats were born. The boys were very obedient around my father, and he liked them, even though he had heard all of the horror stories about their profanity.

Our petite English next door neighbor believed that kindness would prevail in developing a rapport with the "brat brothers." One day, she invited them in for milk and cookies. Afterwards, as they were leaving her yard, they both turned and shouted in unison, "We still think that you're an old bitch."

My father had been the most prophetic, assertively stating, "When the 'brat brothers' start attending school they shall become angels." Unbelievably, his prophesy turned out to be true. But prior to their redemption, those two little buggers could really swear. Not surprisingly, they had foul-mouthed parents with loud voices.

One summer day, Cecil and I were hoeing potatoes in our adjacent lot. Very suddenly, a lady came upon us, well dressed and wearing a large hat that matched her outfit. She smilingly exchanged amenities with Cecil, who introduced her to me, "Gus, this is my mother."

She greeted me warmly and said, "Looks like you lads are busy with gardening chores. Cecil, I just stopped by to say hello, and I am going to go into the house and visit with Lois, Dorothy, and Rita. Is Gordon at home too?"

"Yes, Mother."

As she moved toward the house, I said, "You and Lois look very much like your mother. Are you going to go into the house and join them?"

"No, Gus. I am going to stay with you."

"Cecil, you should join the rest of your family and visit with your mother."

"No, I'll stay out here with you."

I was really surprised at his somewhat blasé attitude; however, I made no comment.

Canada, at that time, was a self-governing dominion with a prime minister as head of government and the king of England as sovereign. The national holiday for the Dominion of Canada was July 1. Shortly after Cecil's mother's visit, we all, including my father, attended a gathering early one evening at a local park to celebrate Dominion Day. The famous Seaforth Highlander's Band performed a medley of their great Scottish tunes. There were other musical artists performing and it was very exciting.

During the gathering, I was standing next to my father when Laura came rushing over to tell my father that our mother was standing nearby and that she had just spoken with her. Laura pointed in her direction and it was the first time I had seen my mother since I had gone into the hospital five years earlier. My father bent his head and whispered to me to go and see her. By this time, she and I had exchanged glances, but she had made no effort to signal that she recognized me or that she wanted me to join her. In my young mind, I thought perhaps she didn't want to see me.

I remained standing by my father until the concert was over and we left. I had ignored my father's pleas to go over and see my mother. With no sign of acknowledgement, I felt too uncomfortable to go on my own. I spent a great deal of time thinking about that incident. I wasn't crestfallen, as she wasn't really part of my life, but I pondered over her behavior, which I considered a slight and a display of her indifference.

Our only mode of transportation in those days was the streetcar service lines. The British Columbia Electric Company provided excellent service throughout the city. There was another Munro family living close to our compound. A blind lady called Agnes resided in their home; she was a switchboard operator at the Blind Institute. Arrangements were made so that Lois could accompany Agnes on the streetcar to and from work each day. In providing this service, Lois received a small stipend and a weekly streetcar pass.

The streetcar fare was seven cents for adults and four cents for children. One adult ticket would cover two children. Lois's weekly pass was truly a gift. Each week the pass would be available to members of the family. Cecil was allocated the pass every other Sunday afternoon and took me with him. We would ride the streetcars from the beginning to the end of the lines—all day long. At the end of the day, we had to come home and report to the family what lines we had taken and if we had seen any interesting sights. This was a great exercise in learning our way around the city.

Both fathers accepted a singular role in outings for our entire family. Lloyd would take the whole family on special picnics during the summer months. We would vote on which of Vancouver's many popular beaches we would visit each time. We kids went to the beaches on our own over the summer months; however, we most enjoyed being there in a family picnic setting. We loved the picnic baskets of food Lois prepared in advance at home.

My father took us to downtown movies, and we would take the streetcar. Lois had her pass, and, aside from my father, there were seven kids. With the movie, along with refreshments, my father tried to be somewhat frugal and he would give the conductor four adult tickets to cover himself and seven others, which was not quite enough even though one adult ticket served for two of the younger kids. In the spirit of the Depression, the conductors always waved my father through despite the shortfall.

However, my father was always irritated because we younger kids would all take separate window seats, instead of sitting together and quietly being inconspicuous. Before we left for movie nights with him, he would always caution us to sit together, but, through our excitement, we would forget and our behavior would usually be table conversation the following night at dinner. Dad would tell Lloyd of his embarrassing streetcar dilemma; we would all laugh, including our fathers.

We had another blind family friend, Ivan, who came to our house on a regular basis. When I was ten years old, Ivan accepted an agreement with St Paul's Hospital to operate a magazine and confectionary stand in their main lobby. In order to get this venture started, Ivan needed to acquire fixtures, equipment, and merchandise from various organizations in downtown Vancouver. For some reason, I was selected to accompany him to the various places of business. This task took place over one summer. He resided in a downtown resident hotel, and I would pick him up in his room on those days when he needed to conduct business. I would arrive at his room, and we would go to the hotel coffee shop so that he could have his breakfast before we started out. Having never eaten in a restaurant, I found the breakfast menu fantastic.

He routinely asked, "Did you have breakfast?" I always said, "Yes." I used to drool at the delicious food served to him, but I was wise enough to realize he was frugal and on a limited budget. During his breakfast, we would review the business trip schedule, and I would learn exactly where we needed to go. Those weekend excursions with Cecil, using Lois's streetcar pass, had substantially increased my adroitness in getting around the city as a precocious ten-year-old.

Arriving home after one of our trips, I was greeted by Lois and Dad who were both sitting in the kitchen getting ready to prepare the evening meal. It was late afternoon, and I asked with hesitancy, "May I have something to eat before dinner?"

Lois inquired, "I assume Ivan took you for breakfast, but you didn't stop for lunch?"

"No—I don't eat at all during our trips."

Dad responded, "Doesn't Ivan usually have his breakfast before starting the day?"

I said, "Yes."

Lois interjected pointedly, "Are you telling us that you just sit and talk with him while he is having his breakfast?"

"Yes. Each time he asks if I would like breakfast and I say, 'No.' Ivan is blind. He needs his money to cover food and rent."

Lois was aghast. "Gus, we'll give you food money every time you go with him." I refused to accept it. Although only age ten, I had an awareness of Ivan and his needs. Lois was always concerned with my wellbeing; she was not too happy to hear that I didn't eat when I was out with Ivan.

She was so concerned that I really felt very special that day. Lois was a very important member in our combined families, and I felt I was very special to her. I had copper-colored hair and a face full of freckles. I hated my appearance and felt very sensitive about it. That day, Lois called me, as a form of endearment, "my little freckled-face Gus."

"I hate these freckles."

Dad chimed in by saying, "I had twice as many as you."

"What? Where did they go?"

He laughed. "They just disappeared."

"Wow, I hope you're right about mine disappearing!"

Lois's final comment was, "Gus, after your evening bath, you look so handsome I always want to squeeze you. And you look so clean!"

"Don't. Cecil will make fun of me."

We three laughed after enjoying a special, quiet moment, separate from the rest of the family—pleasant, but too infrequent.

Ivan was very successful in his business venture and some time later the local newspapers showed pictures of him actually building his own home—with others helping him structurally, of course. He was totally blind and would work on the house after work in the wee hours of the morning. The neighbors complained about the noise and hammering, but I saw him as a truly remarkable human being.

A most unique streetcar service operated in south Vancouver on Main Street, and it ran from 50th Avenue to Marine Drive. There were two streetcars covering that particular line. The two streetcars left simultaneously from opposite ends and met halfway—one pulling over to a sidetrack. They exchanged a stick just as runners do in a relay race. The seats were made of wood and they were reversible—you simply turned the back to face either way. The slang name for this streetcar line was "Hinky Dinky." I had been visiting a Scottish family and, when I departed, the uncle, Big Angus, walked me to the streetcar. (In our clan, we were known, respectively, as Big Angus and Little Angus.)

We saw the Hinky Dinky coming and he gave me five cents to run into the corner confectionary store to get an all-day sucker, which was my favorite. He said to hurry. I got on the Hinky Dinky and waved to Big Angus. Then I opened my sucker to find a coupon entitling me to receive another one for free! This had never happened to me before, but I knew that there was a proviso—one must be in the store when opening the sucker in order to receive the free one. I am a generous and not overly materialistic individual, but in my young mind I felt cheated by not getting that free sucker. Ironically, I still feel cheated to this very day. As a child living in the Depression era, receiving that free offer seemed equivalent to winning a lottery. We kids always waited with bated breath for that freebie slip when we opened our sucker wrapper. Until this incident, none of us had received the slip; and none of us ever did afterwards, either.

Burnaby (a suburb of Vancouver) in those days was very rural. We had very close family friends who lived at Caribou Station, which was near the end of the tramline that ran from the Carrall Street terminal to the Sapperton station in New Westminster. I always enjoyed the tram ride even though most of the scenery was bush and deciduous trees. This family had horses and lived a very country life. We used to swim in the small rivers and hike up the backcountry. In the summertime, they had loads of raspberry canes and the berries were served to us with deliciously hot baking powder biscuits. They were out of this world.

Many European groups such as Czechs and Poles—new immigrant Canadians—held festivals or picnics in that area. As so much of the land was totally undeveloped, groups and individuals often took advantage of the virgin regions. They would clear the bush and build a dance floor. Then they would set up tables and benches. Our friends would take us to these events where there was a lot of folk dancing, singing, food, and fun. They were wonderful people and they welcomed everyone. It seemed that many of our close family friends had moved out of the city, preferring to reside in very rural communities. Most were from farming families, and they possessed sort of a pioneering spirit.

I remember, even nearer to home, in the False Creek Flats, there were wonderful Japanese carnivals prior to the war years. Those events were so festive and beautifully adorned with exotic lanterns and numerous concessions. Many of the ladies were colorfully dressed in Japanese costume.

Lloyd became smitten with a former neighbor. After she and her daughter moved, they frequently would come and spend the weekend at our house. The woman, unfortunately, had a nervous condition—her head and hands would shake mildly but incessantly. Aside from her nervousness she was in good health and functioned well. However, she was not too keen in the work department. She loved to work jigsaw puzzles and could sit and work them for hours, her hands shaking as she tried to fit the pieces into the puzzles.

Because she was basically lazy, and due to her condition, we cruelly named her—behind her back—Mrs. Giggle-Britches!

One Saturday morning, Cecil came running into the house searching for my father. Cecil half-shouted to him, "Mrs. G and daughter are coming toward the house!"

"Oh, no!" responded my father, "Cecil, quick! Tell everyone to hide all of those damn jigsaw puzzles. That's all we need this morning is her sitting on her bottom working puzzles."

We were all screaming with laughter. Dad, a normally soft-spoken person, was really having a fit in anticipation of her visit.

That evening, Mrs. G joined our fathers and other family friends for a night in the pub. In the course of the evening, one of our family friends said, "Tell me, Mrs. Giggle—" His wife immediately interceded and said, "Charlie, I need to speak to you!" Away from the table the wife explained, "That is not her real name!"

When that incident got back to the family, we screamed with laughter! I must confess that Lloyd always took our teasing about Giggle-Britches in good humor, possibly because he was so outvoted.

Eventually he remarried—but to someone else.

3

We all loved going to the movies—especially on Saturday afternoons at the Rio Theater located on Broadway at Commercial Drive. It was five cents for admission, and we got a penny extra to cover three pieces of candy. Cecil and I always went to the movies together, and there was normally no problem in obtaining our allowance of six cents. If no funds were available, I seemed to be the more resourceful in addressing the issue. If the lilacs were in bloom, we would pick the best blooms and I would deliver them to neighbors who knew me. I would inform the recipient that my father suggested we share our flowers with them. The grateful neighbor would give me a dime or so to show appreciation and off we'd go to the movies. Cecil thought I was very ingenious, and so did I. I practiced the same scenario with apples later in the season. In desperation we would grab a few wire hangers at home and sell them to the cleaner's for a penny each. And we did this all on the q.t.

Other than the *Wizard of Oz* and a few Disney movies such as *Snow White*, there were few movies tailored for children—Shirley Temple movies being the exception.

Aside from when my father took us as a family group, going to the downtown theaters was an event for us that usually involved another person or family member. We all loved going to the Beacon Theater on Hastings Street, which featured vaudeville acts along with a couple of "B" or "C" movies. The movies would consist of a detective movie—a Boston Blackie type picture—and a Gene Autry or Roy Rogers western movie. One of my best friends, Billy and his brother and I saw Roy Rogers and Trigger live on stage. We sat in the front row and watched the movies twice in order to see Roy and Trigger on stage a second time.

I always enjoyed going to town with my father. He was six foot four (with pompadour hair that made him look even taller)—one of the tallest men in Vancouver. He had a perfect build and was never a pound overweight. He was an extremely strong, but a very gentle and moral man. People were always greeting him on the street. He was well liked and popular. He would tell me interesting stories about the people we met, but, paradoxically, he was seldom able to recall their names. I felt so important being with him and was pleased to be included when we met people.

I remember one day we stopped for haircuts. My father had given me a quarter to pay the barber. I had my haircut first and, after paying the barber, I slipped the remaining change into my father's hand. He handed it back to me. I said with bewilderment, "But Dad, this is ten cents!"

He whispered, "Keep it!"

My father had a very good friend, an elderly bachelor, who was a clockmaker, and I always loved going to visit him. He had a very small apartment with lots of shelves filled with second-hand mantel clocks, all chiming in unison. He also had old-fashioned standard alarm clocks that ticked noisily, and some pocket watches and wristwatches. I recall that, in his tiny living quarters (and he himself was diminutive in stature), stood a huge wood-burning stove—coal black, with all of the metal parts glistening. In size and appearance it seemed to overwhelm his small apartment. However, his combined work and living quarters were incredibly immaculate.

On one visit, my father casually asked, "Do you have a watch that would be suitable for my son?"

The watchmaker handed me a beautiful watch and said, "Do you like this one, Angus?"

I was completely flabbergasted, but managed to say, "Yes, I love it!"

He and my father both apparently noticed my look of astonishment and laughed.

"Angus," said the clockmaker, "stop by after school tomorrow. I need to adjust the wristband and clean the moving parts."

"Thank you both for this wonderful gift."

It was the longest twenty-four hours I had ever spent. I loved the watch; it had cost my father $2.75. I pondered over the fact that I had been given this wonderful gift, and I tried to comprehend what I had done to deserve it. Materialistically, it was the most treasured gift that I ever received. I kept and used that watch for years and years.

Facing the front of our house and beyond the meadows were the railroad tracks for both the Canadian National Railway and the Great Northern Railroad.

We could clearly see the trains arriving and departing each day. In 1938 and the first half of 1939, the Depression still existed. We would often see dozens of men sitting on top of the freight cars coming to the city. These men would jump from the trains before they reached the station to avoid railroad security guards. Many came to our back door for food, and we did our best to provide for them. My father explained that they were good people simply out of work because of the Depression. Occasionally, one or two remained in the area. One person lived in one of the abandoned railway tool sheds for several months, and he would bring jars and tins to our house for replenishment. We always did our best to help others. Even though we ourselves had a very abstemious lifestyle, we distributed as much as we could to everyone in need.

The Royal Visit of King George VI and Queen Elizabeth took place in 1939. One morning, we were surprised and excited to see the magnificent royal blue train bound for the Canadian National Railway Station. Beyond the railroad tracks was the City of Vancouver garbage dumping ground. The royal visitors would be touring and passing over the First Avenue Viaduct. The city garbage management personnel spent two weeks covering up the dumpsite to eliminate the dreadful smell. We saw the king and queen for the first time there, and it took less than five minutes for them to drive by that carefully prepared site. The king, while exhibiting shyness, looked regally distinguished. And the queen, dressed in royal blue from head to toe, looked so elegant and gracious in manner. Her wave to her cheering subjects was her hallmark. Mundanely, the next day the dump trucks returned back to the dumpsite.

My first train trip took about forty-five minutes. I traveled via the Great Northern Railroad to Alexander's Fresh Air Camp at Crescent Beach. We were there for two weeks and we spent a lot of time at the beach. You could walk seemingly for miles when the tide was out. Boundary Bay seemed almost touchable. One day, I was in a rowboat and we got stuck on the sand bar. I was eleven my last year at camp and I was selected as a representative from my particular camp group.

A Vancouver City alderman and his wife were coming to the camp to bestow certain privileges on those selected campers. Before meeting with them, I had a slight case of influenza that produced severe diarrhea that sent me running frequently to the restroom (a.k.a. the outhouse). When my name was called at the gathering, the alderman informed me that I had been named Health Inspector of the camp. How very appropriate—having the runs and all. I was extremely impressed with the alderman and his attractive wife, as they were a well-groomed and distinguished-looking couple. They were so amiable and made us feel so very important that day.

I saw my first Santa Claus at Spencer's Department Store when I was about five. I saw him after I'd taken a ride on a small train. I could tell that his beard was a fake and I truly never ever believed in Santa Claus. The lad next door to us received many more presents than Cecil and I did. However, I realized he was the only one in the family and could expect more. Christmas was a very realistic experience for me and I was grateful for whatever I received.

The Inglehart family had a special day every Dominion of Canada Day, which is celebrated on the first of July. It was a midyear celebration that honored the previous Christmas, and every member of their family gathered in their father's bedroom while he opened the family trunk. The trunk contained one special and cherished Christmas gift for each member of the family that had been saved from the previous year. Each family member could keep the gift for that day only. All gifts were placed back in the trunk the following day for another year.

It was an exciting celebration for them, and the trunk was a certain form of security for that family. Cecil believed that whatever possessions or funds his father had acquired were concealed in that trunk.

As a combined family, the nicest gift we received every year or so was a new floor-model radio. We all gathered around the radio in the evenings, and especially on the weekends, and listened to our favorite radio programs. I loved all of the ghost and mystery stories. We all seemed to enjoy the same programs. Whether you were eight or eighty, you listened to the *Hit Parade*, and everyone knew the latest songs. My sister Laura, a great dancer, taught us all to do the jitterbug. Laura often appeared in neighborhood concerts as she became well known for her tap dancing. I would resourcefully tell the monitor at the door I was her brother and I should therefore be let in free. I sat inconspicuously alone, as she would know I had fudged my way in by using her name. She was very popular and incredibly beautiful—and a great dancer.

Unless one was really seriously ill, my father always believed one should go to work or school and perform whatever duties or obligations one had been assigned. The mumps had hit our area and one or two members of the family had mild cases.

The school nurse had instructed my sister and me not to attend school until the quarantine date had expired. My father disagreed with those instructions. He said they were ludicrous and told us to go to school. I was in the fifth grade and the school nurse came to my classroom door with my sister, Marjorie. My teacher instructed me to meet with the school nurse outside of my classroom.

"Angus, Marjorie informed me this morning that your father instructed you both to attend classes at school instead of honoring the quarantine period. Is that correct?" Aside from being caught off guard, I was really embarrassed and answered, "Yes!"

"Angus, you must realize that this is a very upsetting situation—you both attending class when other members of your family recently had the mumps. You and Marjorie are to leave school immediately and you are not to return until after the quarantine period. When you return, come to the nursing office before you attend class."

We were three blocks from home and I knew that our father was at home that day and would be angry with my sister for provoking this situation. I said, "Wait till Dad hears what you've been up to."

However, before we reached home, she convinced me that being out of school for a few days should be quite agreeable. I finally concurred and we informed our father that the nurse had pursued us and was upset and demanded we honor the quarantine period. Some sojourn—I got the mumps the very next day and Marjorie got them the following day.

My sister Laura and I were the only two in the family who attended church on Sunday. When I was about nine years old, I was selected to make the church announcements each week pertaining to prayer meetings, choir practice, and other events. The information I needed to convey each Sunday was written on the blackboard in one of the side rooms. Sometimes I wasn't called to make the announcement until near the end of the service, and I often by then had forgotten what I was to announce. Fortunately, the kind and thoughtful minister identified my shortcomings and bailed me out on those occasions when I screwed up. Laura would cringe with embarrassment. I naively thought the minister and I made a great team.

Occasionally, we would have a roster of guest speakers at our church—visiting missionaries mainly from China and Africa—and it was fascinating to listen to their experiences. I was really interested in the missionaries who were stationed in China. During the 1930s, Japan had invaded China and much of their country was under Japanese occupation. The missionaries really opened my mind at an early age, teaching us that we lived in a very volatile world. Living in an age of limited communications, I felt privileged to receive this first-hand information, and, as a child, I really recognized what beneficial services the missionaries performed. The missionaries and my father taught me so much about world affairs at such an early age.

Great Britain and her empire went to war in the fall of 1939. Newsboys were screaming throughout our city that we were at war. We had radio, but, to see any pictures relating to war, we depended on our newspapers and magazines.

World news was shown on movie screens, but not during the children's Saturday matinee. At school the teacher would roll down the world map showing the British Empire and she would review the United Kingdom and all of her dominions and possessions.

When World War II started, Canada was the second largest country in the world in size, but had just over 11,000,000 people. Logistically, most of the country relied on the transportation services of two national railways, the Canadian National Railroad (CNR) and the Canadian Pacific Railway (CPR). The population lived in a very thin ribbon running across Canada, which is well over 3,000 miles in length. Most of the population dwelled one hundred miles or so north of the U.S. border.

The Depression ended in 1939 when World War II started. Many went into military service, and the job market changed from zero jobs available to thousands of positions in industry and commerce. Both men and women worked in the shipyards and other defense plants and other industries, with many persons working two or three jobs during the war years.

In June 1942 our house was sold and the Inglehart family bought a fixer-upper nearby. They said farewell to their chickens and goats—and to us, the Munros. We moved to a rental unit. While these events unfolded, I was absolutely devastated that our families would be parted. Our home, family, goats, chickens, gardens, lilac bushes, and apple trees had been my very existence. Everything I wanted and that was dear to me was in that setting. Everyone else seemed to accept these changes ebulliently, really looking forward to our separate moves.

I felt like an orphan having to return to my former insular existence. I spoke to no one regarding my feelings and knew that nothing good was on the horizon for me. Conversations concerning our separate moves, along with the preparations, sadden me beyond belief. I believe unequivocally, that this separation was more devastating to me than it was to any other member of either family. Our four years together had definitely been the happiest of times for me in my eleven and one-half years.

Aside from home, I was doing very well at school and finished about fourth or fifth in my class out of thirty-six students. I loved my church and all of the missionaries from other lands who came to see us and tell us about events that were happening around the world. I loved going to the Rio Theater each Saturday with Cecil and the others. I loved playing, running, and biking throughout the neighborhood. I enjoyed quiet times on the False Creek meadows traveling "to and fro" with our goats, Molly and Peggy, and stopping to lie in the thick grass and admire the blue sky and clouds! Aside from goat herding, I did my other chores also with alacrity, such as delivering milk, feeding and watering the chickens, gathering their eggs, tending to my rabbits, and doing my gardening. Simplistic stuff, yes, but wonderfully fulfilling to me. My happy life!

4

After we left the Inglehart family, I was soon to learn the stark reality that my happy childhood of the past four years was about to end. It was 1942 and, due to the war, there was a tremendous housing shortage everywhere. My father rented a dilapidated townhouse unit. It was screaming for an exterior paintjob and major repairs or—better still—demolition. Our rent was eight dollars per month. I would take our rent payment along with some of the other neighbors' payments to the widowed owner who resided in the fashionable residential west side of the city. I took the streetcar to the landlady's apartment. She was quite elderly, but very businesslike and always failed to thank me for my messenger service. However, as our rents were so low, and the place in such disrepair, I was certain our units were burdensome for her to have to retain with no management services.

The landlady had a Queen Mary regal look about her. She was matronly in both appearance and dress, and showed a combined demeanor that was gracious but austere. I was never invited into her lavish apartment that appeared so opulent to me. It seemed to be loaded with expensive antiques, both in her furnishings and accessories—certainly a far cry from her rental units. She had an enormous roll-top desk in her hallway at which she prepared individual receipts for my payments. I was never invited in. Remaining at the door awaiting her completion of numerous rent receipts was a slow process. Our conversations were as follows:

"Good morning, Mrs. Mutree. I have some payments for you."

"Hello, Angus, I shall prepare receipts for you."

"Thank you."

"Some of the tenants have not paid their rent, which is very upsetting to me. When your father volunteered your service so that I would not have to come to each unit monthly, I thought that he would check with each tenant on my behalf."

"Mrs. Mutree, my understanding is that I would be available to bring all payments to you if your other tenants paid their rent to my father."

"Angus, your father should address the rent-due issue to those in arrears. Some are paying but they are still behind, and I need them brought up to date."

"Mrs. Mutree, our telephone number is Fairmont 2680L, and I suggest you call my father regarding those unpaid rents."

"I shall call your father and discuss it with him and ask for his assistance."

"Mrs. Mutree, I shall be happy to bring additional rent payments as soon as they have been collected."

"I expect you shall, Angus."

This lady had great dignity and I thought she was very regal and interesting. I felt embarrassed that she had difficulty in obtaining the very low monthly rent payment from some of the other tenants. My father had simply volunteered my delivery services and did not want close involvement in having to confront a couple of the deadbeat renters. My father had no personal responsibility to bang on doors for rent money, as we were just one of the renters, too. And I was merely a youngster, so having to be subjected to all of this "adult stuff" was ludicrous. However, I personally believed the onus should have been with my father to help this elderly lady instead of appearing so lax in his involvement. He actually surprised me with his indifference to Mrs. Mutree's plight. He viewed her as a very wealthy lady. And to me that was not the point. What was due should be paid. It was disappointing to me to see adults not meeting their personal responsibilities and I thought it untenable.

Our apartment was one of eight units located in a predominantly industrial district in Vancouver. Instead of viewing the open meadows, bush and treed reserves of False Creek Flats, I now viewed the West Coast Shipyards. The shipyard was essential to our war efforts, but selfishly I considered it a noisy neighbor, as the shipyard ran three full shifts daily. Their wartime commitment was to launch a merchant ship every six weeks. War bond drives were held in the shipyards, and celebrities would come to promote the annual drive. Being at close range, we were privy to spectator observations.

One year, I saw actress Barbara Stanwyck at touchable range. Another year, comedian Jack Benny and his radio personalities, including Rochester, visited.

Vacancies in our buildings had occurred as Japanese families who had lived in the units for many years were being sent to internment camps in the interior of British Columbia. They were wonderful people, and we were sorry they were forced to leave the coastal area. My father assisted the families in trying to obtain reasonable prices for the furnishings and personal belongings they had to part with before they were sent to their new wartime (and more confining) living quarters. Before the families left, the authorities confiscated certain items such as radios and cameras. Because of the confiscation, my father invited both children and adults to our unit to listen to their favorite radio programs.

The fact that we lived in a household so obviously absent of maternal influence afforded our neighborly Japanese mothers to diligently check the wardrobe of my younger sister. Their examination would reveal what needed to be mended and what buttons needed to be replaced. In performing these tasks, the only proviso was that my father was never to be told for fear that he may be embarrassed by their intervention. The ladies didn't want him to think they thought that he was neglecting his duties. However, my sister was always grateful to these women and expressed her appreciation to my father. Dad was never surprised by their generosity or kind gestures, and always said that one never needed to lock their doors with Japanese neighbors, as they were wonderful, trustworthy people.

My favorite Japanese neighbor was Rosie. She was about twenty, lived with her mother, and was an absolute sweetheart. She really took to our family and considered my father a very honorable man for being so sympathetic and helpful to our Japanese neighbors and their plight. She was so much fun. As they were in a transitional period awaiting resettlement orders, my father hired her services to make curtains and window shades for our entire unit. This enabled her to make a little extra money before leaving Vancouver.

One evening, long after the imposed curfew time, one of our family friends, who was visiting and in the Canadian Army Military Police, was instructed by my father to escort Rosie home, which was five doors down. Vivacious Rosie, who was thoroughly enjoying the evening, facetiously said to my father, "Munro, you could have us all arrested for the detainment of my visit!"

While everyone laughed it was not really funny. Rosie was a wonderful and loyal Canadian, who was faced with insensitivities such as a curfew in her own homeland. After she settled into the "resettlement camp" she wrote a long and cheerful letter stating how beautiful the landscape was in the interior of British Columbia. We treasured her friendship; she had instantaneously become part of our family, as we loved her so.

The resettlement of the Japanese in camps had commenced a few months before we moved in among our Japanese neighbors. The fathers and older sons were taken to the resettlement camps or they enlisted in the Canadian military services.

My father worked at the Hamilton Bridge steel plant that was adjacent to the shipyards to meet the latter's structuring demands. He also held a second job unloading cargo on our busy wartime waterfront. Between the two jobs he was kept busy. He was at Hamilton Bridge a full afternoon shift five days a week and worked days during the week on the waterfront and sometimes full weekends.

Because of the long hours at the waterfront, my dad earned a large amount of overtime benefits, which he loved after the horrible Depression years.

My older sister Laura stayed with us periodically; however, most of the time our household consisted of my father, my younger sister Marjorie, and me. This eleven-year-old—former happy goat herder—out of necessity, quickly learned to accept the responsibility of keeping the house clean, going to the market, and fulfilling all other domestic activities. We had the luxury of having our laundry sent out each week—the laundry did a superb and inexpensive job. It was not a wash-and-fold situation—our bed linens were ironed and our shirts were starched and pressed—they always looked perfect.

My father was a good cook; however, during those years I, too, was responsible for getting the meals prepared, although my cooking skills were definitely substandard. No one had taught me anything relating to domestic duties—including preparing meals. Prior to our separation from the Inglehart family, I could only prepare a cup of cocoa and toast a slice of bread and load it with peanut butter.

According to family, neighbors, and friends, I miraculously learned to consistently prepare a delicious beef stew with dumplings. Virtually, everyone who lived in our complex was aware of my limited culinary skills but came en masse on stew night. They would voluntarily grab bowls from the pantry to enjoy my only contribution that would have been acceptable to an epicure. Aside from my stew and dumplings, I could make great homemade biscuits from scratch.

We did our cooking on a woodstove and my father kept our basement supplied with lumber ends he could freely take from a nearby lumber mill. He carted them home in gunnysacks. I helped in the process, as well, to replenish our wood supply that was essential for daily cooking and for heating hot water and keeping our unit warm.

My father, like so many others, gratefully worked hard and long hours during the war years after experiencing a terribly long Depression and mass unemployment. Although my father was basically soft-spoken, he was an excellent conversationalist on both topical and historic issues, and he presented his views effectively. For a farm boy with a limited education, he was very comfortable and dynamic in conversing with people from all walks of life.

He loved thought-provoking people and knew many successful businessmen and professional people and many local politicians. At that time, William Lyon Mackenzie King was the prime minister of Canada. His early family ties included a close relationship with our Munro family—back East.

The Munros were all descended from early Scottish settlers based in southern Ontario in the early 1800s, engaged in farming. As prime minister, King was not too popular in British Columbia. My father cautioned me never to mention any family association. My father was never a name-dropper—and he was never socially impressed.

My father particularly loved arguing (at his pub club) with the local politicians; however, he remained extremely courteous even when discussing controversial topics. Unlike me, he had extreme liberal views, and we would argue at the breakfast table almost every morning. I was about thirteen when these breakfast conversations commenced and, to his credit, he treated me in an adult manner. He was never ever condescending when I expressed my adolescent opinions. He expected me to keep current on the war news and other issues by reading the newspaper each day. He spoke softly, but commandingly and compellingly. Always assured of his convictions.

My father was a voracious reader, consuming newspapers, periodicals, and books. He read in bed each night during the week for at least an hour. His favorite lighthearted reading included books by American novelist Erskine Caldwell. We shared the same bedroom and, laughing out loud, he would raise his voice and read humorous passages to me. On the aftermath of the Great Depression, on social issues, my father was more in accordance with the works of another American writer, John Steinbeck, whose 1930 writings clearly depicted impoverishment. Dad had an inquiring mind, but unlike me, he maintained strong and passionate liberal beliefs.

My father could easily vindicate his plight caused by his experience of mass unemployment during the Depression. He failed to address some of his personal shortcomings relating to his earlier years in farming. He had had his wealthy father's support in getting him both stabilized and permanently established. Any conversation relating to either my grandfather or my dad's brother Uncle Earl was normally of a very negative nature. Although it was never discussed, I perceived that my father remained heartbroken over being excluded from his father's will.

Dad's brother Earl was a diabetic, and the state of his health was somewhat precarious. Additionally, treatment in those days was obviously limited. Shortly after we separated from the Inglehart family, a telegram was delivered to our unit. I opened it and found it to be from my uncle's widow, informing us that he had passed away due to his diabetic condition. He had been only in his late thirties.

My father was working two jobs and he telephoned to check in with us. I informed him of the telegram and read the message. He replied, "Don't wait for me for dinner. I'll be working late." He had been so crestfallen over his brother's behavior regarding his father's will there was no longer an emotional attachment.

When we were alone, my father often spoke with me regarding the various members of his family. He absolutely adored his mother, and one sister was special to him. While he complimented both his father and brother on their positive traits, he overall had very negative feelings for both. Frankly, he never related to them.

I assumed my father inwardly believed that his father always favored his brother. And that may have been true because of my dad's rebellious nature. He clearly stated that his father was the most respected farmer in the community and considered the wealthiest. He had other very wealthy relatives as well—all from successful farming families. I was impressed by his comments regarding our family in eastern Canada, who had remained on their original property.

He said of his grandfather, whom he had seen only in his very early childhood, "He was extremely hardworking and wealthy, but very outgoing and loved parties and was very charismatic and enjoyed socializing. They had their own Scotch whiskey still on their vast farmlands in Ontario. He was my kind of guy—more lighthearted and unlike my austere disciplinary father." He said, "He was just like me and loved parties and fun, while my father was all work and no play."

He also said, "My father informed me that in every other generation we get a dud—meaning me, of course." Then he continued, "Gus, you favor your grandfather and I favor mine!"

"Do you really think so, Dad?"

"I see you in 'my old man' in so many ways, and he would have loved you. Two peas in a pod."

Both of my father's parents expired before I was born and I loved hearing stories about them. However, I made my own assessments, many based from my own personal observations as well as from hearing unbiased stories from other relatives and old family friends who helped me form my own conclusions.

My grandmother was from a Scottish-American hotel family who originally settled in Pennsylvania in the 1830s, and they had been moderately successful.

Even at my young age, I surmised that, in terms of our Munro family and heredity, we had had a very impressive hardworking agrarian background. My father, with his impulsive and rebellious nature, just didn't seem to fit that mold.

It was very clear to me that members of my Scottish family, after arriving in Canada, were truly pioneers and contributed greatly in developing their land holdings in both in Ontario and Saskatchewan. As a child, I tried to find my identity through my father. It was impossible, as we had such divergent interests. He was totally non-materialistic and only wanted to remain debt free, and to hell with any acquisitions. Although I mildly have been somewhat subdued materialistically, I viewed our family as the "riff raff" among our other relatives, with my father as head honcho. I kept those thoughts shamefully to myself.

Dad's mind worked so quickly, an elocution teacher would have pulled the reins to slow down his speech. In meeting him, one of my friends said, "He speaks so quickly, I picked up only half of his conversation." That friend later went on to build several skyscrapers in Vancouver and western Canada and was certainly no dummy. Despite his shyness, everyone truly loved my father. He set a high moral standard and he was tremendously respected and an extremely generous person. Young and old seemed to quote him and espouse his political views without question—with the exception of myself. Deep down I believe he admired my rebelliousness and my willingness to express my divergent political views.

One evening, my father was engaged in a lengthy telephone conversation. My sister returned home during this period and asked who my father was speaking with on the telephone. As a young kid and most definitely prone to high jinks, I nonchalantly responded by saying, "Oh, probably some old bag."

My father, still on the telephone, made no mention of my stupid comment. About a week later, I arrived home from school to find my father sitting in our kitchen having late afternoon tea with a very attractive woman. As soon as I approached the kitchen with inquisitive anticipation, my father stood up and smilingly said, "Gus, this is the old bag I was speaking with over the telephone last week."

Fortunately, the lady projected herself delightfully and laughingly and very graciously introduced herself, her behavior virtually calming me from embarrassment. She was visiting from Washington State and was a kin of close family friends. She was happy to participate with my father in teaching me a lesson.

My father thought I had a great sense of humor in commenting on some of our eccentric acquaintances. He found my comments outrageously amusing and subtlety accurate. He, therefore, liked to reciprocate at every opportunity.

After living apart from the Inglehart family, with my father working two jobs, we became fairly well off financially. Aside from my dad's spendthrift lifestyle, his Scottish background would occasionally become prevalent, as he was adamant in being totally debt free. He never ever charged anything and purchased only what he could pay for in cash. At Christmastime, he would ascertain what friends or neighbors we knew had experienced a difficult financial year. He would share his Christmas work bonus with those persons and also arrange to spend Christmas with a family in need.

One year he shared his Christmas bonus with a neighbor whose husband had abandoned her, leaving her pregnant and with two small children. I must add that the estranged husband was strong on brawn but weak in responsibilities in caring for his family. One evening, he had picked up our large solid oak dining table with his teeth only and lifted it three feet in a balanced position. He demonstrated outstanding strength; however, he turned out to be a weakling in providing for his family.

When arranging the Christmas dinner, my father would telephone a family, temporarily in need, suggesting we spend Christmas together, stipulating it should be at their home. He would state that he had two hungry kids and that he didn't plan on spending the day cooking just for our small family. He would mention that we would be bringing a turkey and a ham donated by his employer along with other food items and some bottles of dinner wine. His request for an invitation with these needy friends was always graciously received and appreciated. These were always very festive and happy events. However, we were notably cautioned individually to never ever discuss my father's holiday season generosity with anyone.

Because of my father, our apartment was equivalent traffic-wise to a mini Grand Central Station. On the weekends, in the breaks in his work schedule, he held parties or poker games, both of which usually lasted all night. I state facetiously that I was afforded the privilege of cleaning up the mess in the aftermath of those events. I personally rapidly developed a deep-seated resentment toward my father and his lifestyle. I did not enjoy the exposure and sharing my life and home on an ongoing basis with dozens of his neighbors, co-workers, acquaintances, and friends. During the week, while he was home, we rarely seemed to be without company. There were occasions when family friends or people from out of town would come and stay with us for various reasons until they got reconnected elsewhere.

Everyone loved coming to our house for parties and fun. Musicians and other talented people loved to come and play their musical instruments or sing and dance. Many came on a regular basis and/or on a moment's notice. My father enjoyed being surrounded with talented individuals who added so much to his parties. For a basically shy person, he had a magnetic charm and he always appeared to be in the middle of everything. He would meet entertainers in his pub club and they would come to the house and perform for us.

We met some exciting and forthright talented people, along with a few licentious bums. The "bums" came opportunistically, to ingratiate themselves with the womenfolk. Strangely, I had an innate talent in quickly identifying the lotharios that we discreetly gave the "bum's rush" in terms of future parties when my morally straitlaced father accepted my observations. He thought I was blessed with an uncanny perception of new people who arrived at our home. He was the active participant, and I was the constant subtle observer with a proven track record—which he found to be indisputable.

My father had a nice singing voice, but he was too shy in public or even at our house parties to sing. When we were alone at home, I really enjoyed hearing him sing western and country music. At parties, my sister Marjorie and I were always called to jitterbug for the group. We always seemed to be a hit but, frankly, we didn't dance well together. Laura taught me ballroom dancing, but I was totally out of her league. It was a teacher-and-student situation and she was a hard taskmaster and a perfectionist.

5

One of our neighbors had a polished operatic voice and both she and her daughter were always a hit singing semi-classical and classical music at our parties. The mother was a Caucasian, but she also spoke Punjabi, as her husband was from India. She cooked the most wonderful variety of East Indian dishes. She taught me to make various curry dishes. They later moved to another district. When she came to our house to visit, we always made certain to have the necessary ingredients for her to prepare the meal. It was a forgone conclusion that she would superbly prepare supper. She had a great sense of humor, was pleasingly plump, and at parties always started her repertoire with *Madame Butterfly*. Initially, as a precursor, she would stand in the middle of the room, and melodiously and in somewhat of a bellowing manner sing, "I'm as free as the breeze and I can do as I please, open song, open road!"

Sometimes we held parties at her home because she had a piano, the playing of which complemented guests who played string instruments. In arranging a forthcoming party at her home my father once said, "Bea, I have a very talented piano player from my club coming to our next party. He's single—try and dig someone up for him."

She said, "Fine."

On the night of the party, after seeing the piano player's blind date, my father quietly said to Bea, "When I said to dig someone up, I didn't mean literally."

Bea responded, "Short notice, but, after seeing the piano player, a good match."

Bea and Dad had a cordial verbal sparring relationship. My father, intellectually interested, once asked Bea, "What are the topics of conversation when East Indian women gather together?"

She answered, "They normally discuss who got laid the night before."

After hearing about this conversation from my father, I used to laugh to myself any time I saw her with East Indian women. I must add that they were homemakers and non-professional women and they were usually very thin, very attractive, and always colorfully dressed in their native saris.

Bea's daughter Noreen was a beautiful Eurasian whose operatic voice was better trained than that of her mother. She had appeared as a performer in some local concerts and other functions with her beautiful soprano voice. She and I were the same age and had a brother-and-sister type of relationship. We teased each other all of the time and vowed we would never ever marry each other when we grew up. We were like family.

We had one friend who had been an officer in the U.S. Navy. He had been stationed at Pearl Harbor and witnessed that day of infamy, December 7, 1941. He apparently left the service shortly thereafter and moved to Canada.

He was extremely entrepreneurial in negotiating major sales and he had the ability to accumulate vast sums of money. The downside was that he would reach a high point, then go on a binge and squander all of his funds, then sober up, rejuvenate himself, and start the cycle over again. He invariably hit our house on the downslide. My father, whom he adored, was sympathetic and blamed the bombings at Pearl Harbor as the source of his problems and his inconsistencies.

We would nurture him back to health and off he would go. On one episode he brought his love interest with him and we had both him and her to contend with, getting them briefly through another rehabilitation session. His lifestyle was like a teeter-totter—up and down. In those days everyone seemed less sophisticated in trying to comprehend human characteristics, and usually described such patterns of behavior mundanely with one-liners.

A young couple—probably in their mid-thirties—attended some of our parties. I cannot correlate how they came to be included in our large circle of friends. They always sat next to each other and very quietly enjoyed being there. Aside from their quietness, they were both very pleasant and well mannered.

They had two small sons, but we never met the lads, as the couple came to parties rather than family social visits. All social contact with this couple had exclusively been in our home. After a couple of years, we were shocked to learn that the wife had had an affair, and her husband retaliated by becoming an axe murderer—with his wife as the victim.

The husband received a life sentence in prison. There is an old maxim to watch out for the quiet ones—in this case both of them, but for different reasons. It was unbelievable and horribly tragic, and we grieved for their boys who were left parentless.

The parties and social events in our home were always well attended and amusing and fun. My father would not tolerate bad behavior and carefully watched liaisons. For some reason, three ladies—proud members of the local Salvation Army Women's Division—arrived during one of our parties. They were teetotalers; the consumption of alcohol was very disdainful to them. My father, who was usually the center of attention rather than an acting host, when seeing these uniformed ladies, was somewhat curious and attempted to ingratiate himself with them. He offered to make them tea or coffee or, alternatively, other refreshments. They sternly rejected his hospitality. He came by shrugging and whispering to me something like, "I don't know who they are, but I can't please them." He was actually crushed by their unfriendly behavior. This was a true anomaly for him, a social paragon, to experience. They were obviously not party crashers—but poopers. We never ascertained from whence they came.

Our home was considered the "in place" for many years and everyone wanted to attend our parties and poker sessions. With the exclusion of the ladies from the Salvation Army, my father's friends and acquaintances enjoyed fun parties and games. When party overflows occurred, we had to use the next-door unit, mainly for dancing. In other words, we were one big happy extended family.

For me though, I grew more resentful of the ongoing janitorial services of cleaning up after the parties and poker games when everyone left—or sometimes should have left but lingered on. No one—family or visitor—offered to help me, ever.

After the orderly, Spartan but tranquil years with the Inglehart family, I could never accept the following years with my father. I fully understood our motherless existence. I willingly accepted family responsibilities in terms of fulfilling household assignments and being partially responsible for my younger sister during those years. However, I was extremely unhappy existing in a confusing and unstable atmosphere. I was young, and my childhood years seemed to have vanished quickly. I found myself in a proverbial vacuum. By nature, I was not a social creature.

When I was in the seventh grade, one of the students informed the teacher that her fountain pen was missing.

The teacher told the class of this incident and asked, "Does anyone know the whereabouts of the missing pen?" No one responded.

This took place in our home classroom and, at the end of that period, we moved to another classroom for the following subject. At the end of that class we returned to our home classroom. Upon our return, the teacher announced that she had had the students in the other class search each desk for the missing pen. Pointing to me she said, "Angus, the missing pen was found in your desk."

I was absolutely shocked beyond belief and totally devastated. I was pulled out of class and taken to see the principal for my supposed misdeed. I was shattered at being confronted and incredulous that the missing pen had been found in my desk. However, I reacted contentiously and stated unequivocally that I knew nothing of the incident.

Angrily I responded, "If you don't believe me and pursue this further, I'll call my father in and you'll be responsible for the consequence."

While I did not normally practice impoliteness, I was dumbfounded at being placed in such an untenable position with the assumption that I was mendacious in denying the act.

However, in fairness to the teacher, it did look bad for me because the pen had been found in my desk. The situation was bizarre and unfolded so suddenly that I was in a state of semi-confusion. Ironically, regardless of the circumstances, pens were of no interest to me.

The teacher and I returned to the classroom; I was infused with embarrassment. At the end of the day, after leaving class, the lad who sat in the desk behind me, accompanied by three or four other lads, informed me, "Angus, I saw Johnny slip the pen in the open side of your desk just before we changed classes." Johnny's desk was right in front of mine.

He and the other lads were very upset, but had made no attempt to come to my rescue during the inquisition.

I confronted the other boy the following morning, "Did you slip that pen in the side of my desk?"

Said he very sheepishly, "No, I would never do something like that to you."

He and I had been casual pals and he vehemently denied any wrongdoing. I was so bewildered, but could not be accusatory, regardless of what had transpired. I had been falsely accused and, aside from the other lads' claims, the damage had been done. All of the lads in the classroom knew that I had not stolen the pen; however, the girls in the class looked at me very disdainfully and accusatorily. I can only assume that the homeroom teacher and principal both thought I was the culprit, too. I simply did not know and was really too immature to rationalize the situation. I did strongly believe that stealing from others was a heinous crime. And that made the situation even more demeaning to me.

Frankly, I never ever got over that horrible incident. As a person who cherishes honesty and integrity, I could not understand why I had been subjected to that unpleasant situation. It was never ever resolved and I could not seek vindication. Some would view this incident as a childhood mishap; however, to me it was an unfair tragic experience that I should have never encountered. With the situation unresolved, my only response was to "play sick" and miss as much of school as I possibly could. I spent zero time ever studying thereafter. I failed and had to repeat that grade the following term. Thought I, *Who cares?* Sensitively, I was unsuccessfully and desperately trying to hide this unwarranted traumatizing event in my young life.

My personal life was insular and I truly believed that I walked down the road alone. That incident profoundly and with supreme importance took a tremendous toll on me. To make the situation worse, I had loathed that school from the day I started. I hated both my home and school. There was no consoling force and no one ever recognized my sad predicament. I quietly prayed for guidance.

We never had a moment to ourselves at home and yet, paradoxically, I lived a very lonely life: a full house—but empty! My only solace was escaping to movies, whenever possible, or taking long walks.

I always enjoyed speed walking, and I would walk for miles. I especially found walking invigorating after a rainstorm, which were commonplace in Vancouver. I also enjoyed track sports and I could run like a deer, probably from all that running I'd done while rounding up our goats during my earlier childhood.

I can only reiterate that I was very disappointed in and disapproving of my father and his lifestyle, while everyone else thought him to be the greatest person. His time for listening to any of my personal concerns was zero—any effort on my part to talk to him was wasted. I felt totally alone and I constantly questioned my negative thoughts. I was in an ongoing turmoil as everyone loved being with him and loved his generous nature and he was a very bright and interesting person. As an end result, I was continuously faced with my aloneness, and I lacked direction. I was unable to express my feelings to anyone—no one recognized that I was living in a proverbial fishbowl. Those years were sometimes very stimulating and at other times so painful that I cannot express them in words.

After shamefully failing and repeating the seventh grade, I dropped out of school at age fourteen. My employment options, needless to say, were somewhat limited. And I had to think on my own about where to start. I applied for a job as a busboy at the Hotel Georgia. In order to be hired, I had to fib about my age, as no youth was to be hired under the age of fifteen. As I was very tall, my age was never questioned. At that time, the Georgia was the second-largest hotel in Vancouver and was located less than a block from the Hotel Vancouver, the largest. I was actually assigned to the banquet and ballroom catering functions; however, I also assisted in the main dining room and coffee shop when needed. In the banquet rooms, each function required special table settings, and I could never remember from one event to the other what needed to be fulfilled. I soon learned that working in food service was not my forte. But what was?

However, at the hotel we received gratuitous meals in conjunction with our remuneration ($18 per week with no tips involved). I was a tall, very skinny, bottomless pit and the food was both abundant and delicious.

When I started working, they also hired several high school and college students who were out of school for the summer months. In comparison, I quickly relegated myself to the bottom of the educational totem pole. I became an observer rather than a participant. The exception was David, who had just completed high school and was starting university in the fall. He immediately befriended me and realized I was just a little kid among the summer hires.

David had a great sense of humor and we teased each other constantly, but simultaneously got our work done, too.

He was very handsome and all of the young ladies—students and full-time employees—were crazy about him. He epitomized what I wanted to be. He seemed to me a bright student from a stable family, extremely popular, and with no conceitedness. While I admired him, I knew I was too young and totally out of his league. I felt no jealousy, just envy. He invited me to his home and he asked me to do some socializing. I realized I was a fourteen-year-old dropout and that I had nothing to contribute in terms of a friendship. Everyone at the hotel thought I was fifteen and, in practicality, would account for nothing more.

One day, during a laughing spell, he told me very seriously, "You're the nicest little kid I have ever known. Do you realize the sense of humor you have for your age? You're so much fun! I really look forward to working with you every single day. You're definitely my best pal here, Gus"

"Thanks, David. I wish I had your popularity! All the girls here love you."

One day I overheard a conversation, between David and our supervisor. "David, Gus is too young to be working. He should still be in school."

"No—he's just out of school for the summer."

"You're wrong, David. He is not returning to school. I know that for a fact."

"Oh no! I really like Gus. He's so funny and really a very bright lad for fifteen."

"Don't say anything to him. Let's just wait and see what happens, David."

"Okay."

I kept that overheard conversation to myself. They didn't know I was a fourteen-year-old. For a slightly older contemporary, David was a great role model for me; however, I was green with envy. I felt inferior and a loner—a misfit. My self-esteem was deeply submerged in self-doubt and I justified that feeling, knowing I was a school dropout.

At the hotel, many wedding receptions were held in the plush York Room. At one wedding reception, while performing my duties, I noticed two former classmates, Gloria and Barbara, from the school I had attended when we lived with the Ingleharts. We three were the same age—near fifteen. I had had a silent crush on Gloria at school. They were in formal dress and I wore my white service jacket and black slacks and looked quite presentable as a hotel employee. They were both elated to see me and spent most of the evening inconspicuously in my company. They didn't want me to get into trouble for spending too much time with them.

I felt visually rather dapper that evening; however, I realistically knew that their lifestyle was not akin to mine and, above the superficiality, I felt very despondent and inferior. I carried my boyhood crush for Gloria, but knew that a relationship would be hopeless. (She had the most beautiful blue eyes.)

My sister Laura had informed me where our mother was living. She had remarried and had a daughter. I decided to pay her a visit. It was during the day, and she immediately identified me and invited me in. She had long retained the memory of our last meeting at the park where no recognition was acknowledged.

She informed me that she had been in an untenable position as a nosy neighbor had come with her. Her neighbor was unaware of her past experiences, so my mother had put discreetness before recognition that particular evening. I accepted her explanation and truly appreciated the fact that she brought it to my attention after expressing basic amenities.

I noticed that, at every opportunity, my mother made derogatory comments and sly innuendoes about my father. Knowing the circumstances and the outcome and the responsibilities that I had had to accept, I did not graciously receive those comments. And frankly, she didn't even know me. My inner uncomplicated thought was, *The old man comes home after being rejected by his brother and finds you in bed with some cheater. End of story.*

To the contrary, my father never ever demeaned my mother even though we were aware of the circumstances. My observation was that she presumed my father had made critical accusations about her behavior that were totally erroneous. Many of her comments pertaining to my father were mendaciously stated and verifiably so. However, I chose to rise above it all, as I realized she and I would never have an endearing relationship. For my entire life since that horrible evening at age three, I had had only a single parent. My mother, by circumstance, had totally been excluded from my life. On that visit, I tried hard to build and strengthen our relationship; however, I realized that it would never materialize beyond a superficial level. It was too late—no solidification was possible.

My mother was an attractive lady—tastefully dressed, immaculately groomed, and impeccably mannered. In a social setting, she looked superb and quite stunning. She did not have Laura's great beauty, but she was a close runner-up.

She and my father were a total mismatch. I was keenly aware of his shortcomings. Instead of trying to circumvent the past, I was constantly listening to all of her diatribe directed at my father. My youthful observations alerted me to the fact that I simply got stuck with parents who presently required no kudos from me nor would they ever be forthcoming. Another commonality they shared was the fact that each one, during a very quiet moment, expressed love for me and told me how special I was to him or her. Without comment I returned nothing. I did not acknowledge their endearing messages. I truly resented them both for different reasons. I kept my thoughts to myself. When the water deeply flows under the bridge, there is little time for bullshit or gullibility.

My mother stopped by the hotel one day to see me, and everyone thought she was too young to be my mother. She had just turned thirty-five and looked years younger. In her life beyond our family, I would give her performance four stars. She was a wonderful mother to her daughter and an excellent wife to her husband. Her home was immaculately kept and she had gifted culinary skills. They had a very fulfilling and happy life. Her past was a pile of ashes that did not need to be rekindled and stirred.

The world champion heavyweight boxer Joe Louis was a guest at our hotel. I was happy to learn that vanilla ice cream was a menu favorite of his—and mine too. We in Canada loved Joe Louis. We listened intently to his fights on the radio, rooting for him. I wanted to meet him at the hotel but it didn't happen. Busboys received no privileges, but I knew he would have been gracious to me.

There was also a wonderful waitress who worked in the coffee shop at the hotel. We in the catering service worked the evenings and I often, at shift's end, went to my locker room about the same time as this waitress.

She had gorgeous red hair and would always sing "Jesus Loves Me" and perform a little modified striptease number in the hallway, en route to her locker room. She was very subtle. She was a sweetheart with a fantastic sense of humor and she was blessed with a gorgeous figure. And, as demonstrated by her persona, she was anything but reclusive. I was nearly fifteen years old and she was about thirty-five. She loved to tease me—literally speaking—with her Gypsy Rose Lee impression. She was a true lady with class, even with her teasing, sense of humor, and gorgeous figure. She had top billing on my admiration list. She certainly knew I was just a "wet-behind-the-ears" brat. But I loved her antics.

I became more disenchanted and restless at home. Therefore, I impulsively decided to leave the hotel—and Vancouver. My sister Laura and her boyfriend, who were living in Regina, Saskatchewan, were going to spend Christmas in Calgary, Alberta. I decided to meet them there without taking any precautionary steps or establishing any game plan.

I purchased my train ticket and, before departing, I, with slight trepidation, called my father to say good-bye. He knew nothing of my quitting my job or leaving Vancouver. I called home. "Dad, I've quit my job at the hotel and I'm going to Calgary tonight by train."

"What the hell are you talking about?"

"I'm tired of working at the hotel. I'm meeting Laura and her mate in Calgary. They'll be there for the Christmas holidays."

He screamed, "Gus, you get your ass home right now."

Quietly, I responded, "Sorry, I'm leaving. I'm happy to be going to Calgary and work out some plans with Laura."

"You come home right away or you'll be in serious trouble. You're too young to be going anywhere! I expect you to return home this evening without fail. I will talk with you about this entire situation and why you quit your job. Get on the streetcar or a taxi and return home now."

He was absolutely furious and screamed at me for the first time ever. I was unabashed. I thought, *To hell with him.* I was happy to be leaving. I was so young and naive; I saw my future as an adventure. I did not have a care in the world—I felt free at last and inwardly excited. After purchasing my train ticket I had exactly $27 to my name.

6

When I arrived in Calgary, I was shocked at how cold the climate was after the mild weather in Vancouver. I had a couple of days to wait before my sister was to arrive, and I checked into a nice downtown middle-class hotel unquestioned and spent two days going to movies. Unlike my father, who had been upset at my leaving, both my sister and her boyfriend laughed hysterically that I was off to see the world on $27. However, by prudent calculation, my largess had been sufficient to cover my hotel, meals, and movies until my sister arrived.

The boyfriend, a rugged-looking Irish Canadian, was a few years older than my sister and sort of a nefarious character—he seemed a borderline underworld type of guy to me. Laura was beautiful and, unfortunately, had a proclivity to be attracted to underworld-type characters and probably vice versa. I was never street smart and naively never understood those with questionable backgrounds. He was great with me. He laughingly and humorously teased me incessantly.

Ironically, his family was very respectable, and he and my sister came from Regina to spend Christmas with his brother and wife. She was the daughter of a prominent magistrate in Calgary and the epitome of sophistication. He was great and appeared quite polished.

We had a wonderful Christmas with them and they were so gregarious and extremely outwardly kind to this runaway brat. After Christmas and Boxing Day we three departed for Regina. (I am certain Laura called my father surreptitiously and told him not to worry and that she would be responsible for my safety.)

The boyfriend was working in a club in Regina during the winter, and I stayed with them for a few days and visited with a distant relative while there. The boyfriend had concessions with a carnival show that ran during the late spring and summer months. The road show would travel to the municipal district fairs in the provinces of Manitoba, Saskatchewan, and western Ontario, staying at each location for a couple of days. The owner provided all of the transportation, such as trucks and buses. The boyfriend produced and solely performed an animal act that featured rattlesnakes and Texas bull snakes. He also was a partner in a popcorn concession. It was decided that I would spend the summer with them operating the popcorn stand. Thus, we had a plan in place.

My precocious sister had traveled extensively throughout Canada and had visited with many of our relatives. She put a visitation plan together for me to stay with my Munro relatives in Saskatchewan and carry on to visit my McClurg relatives—my mother's side of the family—in Manitoba. The visitation plan was spread over the few months I had free before I had to rejoin my sister and her mate to work with them on the road show. I didn't have a clue as to the logistics of the visitation plan, and didn't know any of my relatives, but I was naively very excited.

It didn't occur to me what type of a reception I would receive from them—me being a skinny, fifteen-year-old, unknown runaway brat at their doorstep.

From Regina, I traveled by bus to visit my father's sister and family who resided in a small town that catered to a farming community. My uncle was a Presbyterian minister and was prominently known throughout Saskatchewan. He and my aunt and family greeted me warmly in their beautiful large home. My uncle had recently returned from serving as a chaplain in the Canadian army overseas. While in wartime London, he had been invited to Buckingham Palace and, along with several other military clergy, had been served tea with the king and queen, followed by cocktails. Their oldest son, Munro, had also just returned from serving with the First Canadian Paratroopers, who had landed in Normandy on D-Day. Munro had been wounded soon after landing in France and found himself being awakened by an attending nurse in an English hospital. Fortunately, he had made a successful recovery. Munro was their only birth child, and they had adopted six other children. Happily, and with the war over, I immediately bonded with this reunited family and they with me.

My aunt quickly perceived my penchant for her wonderful culinary skills—especially her pastries. She informed me that she loved to bake but hated the cleanup chores. Without further ado, she baked and I did the cleanup. I think she correctly surmised that I was not used to having these wonderful treats. Our cooking at home was extremely plain—devoid of pastries, but with quality meats and loads of vegetables and fruits. My father was strong on good nutrition.

They also had an ice cream maker in their cold climate, and I learned to use it and did so virtually every day. To reciprocate, I made some East Indian dishes for the family—all curries. I considered chicken curry my specialty and I received laudatory comments. Truthfully, I had very limited culinary skills.

The family took me to their local ice-skating rink. This awkward Vancouverite tried unsuccessfully, but very earnestly, to learn to skate.

They had a huge organ, and my aunt was very accomplished. I learned that other members of her family had been very musical while growing up. My aunt and uncle were concerned about my being away from home. I sort of intimated that I would just be gone a few months and return home by next fall. They were also concerned about my sister Laura being with a young man and not married, and her mate having a somewhat precarious background. That lifestyle was not too prevalent. Laura had been to their home previously and all members of their family had been captivated by her good looks, meticulous dress, and charming personality. She spoke beautifully and had excellent writing skills and penmanship. I think those skills were beneficial in preparing my visitation plan, as all of my relatives greeted me very warmly and, surprisingly, without question.

I learned from my aunt that, when growing up in Saskatchewan, my father had regularly helped families who were plagued with fatal communicable diseases. My aunt stated that my father was not fearful of the exposure in caring for these rurally isolated families who were faced with this tragedy.

She said he volunteered his services as a teenager and a young man to help with their daily chores and to prepare meals. Additionally, he helped to nurse these families during their horrible plight without regard of his own safety. In many cases, several family members died and he had to actively participate in carrying out those sad burial missions. He had been commendable in assisting the families, but he rarely, if ever, mentioned the subject to me.

My aunt told me, "He was rebellious by nature, but he was courageous. He displayed strong Christian values and convictions starting very early in his youth. Angus, I truly love your father. He is a great person and he freely gave his time to help those in distress in our farming community when we were growing up."

"Yes, he helps those in need in Vancouver, too."

"Your father's rebelliousness toward our father was constant in his childhood."

"I assumed as much."

"One day, several visitors from the community came to visit at our farm. Your grandparents were arranging a special luncheon for them. Your father was very funny. He said, 'Due to my standing, I may as well just join the pigs for lunch.' There was a big water hole in the pig enclosure so he jumped in and started to splash water and mockingly imitated the pigs. 'Oink, oink,' he squealed. My sister, brother, and I watched his performance and laughed hysterically—he was so mischievously funny."

Laughingly I said, "I never heard that story before." I asked her whom she had supported—her father or her brother—in terms of their estranged relationship.

"Your father—my brother—Angus."

I found that interesting, having heard her perceptive comments about my father.

My uncle told me another humorous story that my father had never mentioned. My uncle said that my father was driving by a farm where he noticed that the husband and wife were physically in battle. My father jumped out of his wagon and ran to assist the poor wife by getting in between them. Unfortunately, his Good Samaritan act did not pay off, as both husband and wife in unison started battling with *him*. He decided to make a quick departure and thereafter pledged against intervention in domestic squabbles.

I spent a few weeks with my ministry family. My sister had arranged for my next visit to be with an aunt who was the widow of my father's brother. She had since remarried. She had one daughter, who, in appearance, strongly favored me. They lived in my father's hometown, having leased all of my grandfather's property to other farmers. It was so cold that I never had the opportunity to see my father's childhood home and farmland. I was very disappointed, but it was too cold for me to travel even by sleigh because I didn't have the proper winter warm clothing.

While I visited, the family had been invited to the home of the mayor of this small community. I was greeted warmly, and the mayor spent most of the dinner hour praising my grandfather and his entrepreneurial attributes.

After dinner, as we were entering their living room, their son, who had just returned from the war, pulled me aside. He said he really liked my father and said to send his regards to him. He laughingly recalled seeing my father walking down the street on the way to the pool hall at about forty below zero with an open shirt. Everyone else was wearing a heavy winter neck scarf. He said he really admired my father, whom he thought was so strong and so tough he could weather any storm—nice comments from a soldier just returning from the European Theater.

It seemed to me that my father's brother Earl had lacked some of my dad's brawn; however, according to my aunt (his wife), he had been the handsomest young man in the district. He had been musically very talented and played the violin. Aside from being a ladies' man and highly sought after by the womenfolk, he had also been a practical joker. According to one story, he once approached one of his tough farm guy friends and informed him that another mate—one of equal stature—had informed my uncle that he could beat the crap out of my uncle's mate with one arm. My uncle then convoyed the same story to the other guy, reversing the circumstances. The two tough farm boys were furious and out for blood as they sought each other for battle. They met and collided, and, during the ruckus, one of the guys started quoting my uncle. Suddenly, they halted in the midst of the fight and compared notes and realized that my uncle had instigated the whole thing.

They decided to unite and went looking for the culprit to teach him a lesson. My quick-thinking uncle, seeing them and surmising the situation, was so skillful and articulate that he had both of the tough guys screaming with laughter over the entire situation he had trumped up. They said my uncle had a great sense of humor and he loved to instigate these types of situations—and worm his way out. My remarried aunt spoke sadly of my uncle in glowing terms.

During my visit, my aunt informed me that my father had a very wealthy widowed aunt who lived in another town, nearby. Possibly seeking future legacy considerations for me, she gave me her name and address and suggested I write to her. To placate, I sent her a letter. She responded quickly (at my aunt's address) and must have been quite elderly, as she thought the letter was from my father, not me. I decided it best to just leave it as was and did not reply.

After a visit of two or three weeks with my uncle's widow and family, I went by train to northern Manitoba to visit my mother's parents. While on the train and getting close to the Swan River district where my grandparents lived, I was sitting with an elderly man from there. He knew my grandparents and I explained that I had sent a telegram to them that morning from Winnipeg. As they lived in the country, and were without a telephone, the passenger was certain they hadn't received it. He turned out to be correct and a Good Samaritan. When we arrived at the station we met a young man who also knew our family. He informed the older man that he would take me to my grandparents.

It was late at night and the young man, Russell, took me to his sister's home in town to provide me with some warm winter traveling clothes. Russell's sister was very kind to me, despite the fact that she had recently been jilted by my air force uncle, who was soon to return home with a new bride. My grandparents lived twelve miles out of town and it was decided that I should stay the night at Russell's home. His home was six miles out of town, and we traveled in his horse-drawn sleigh. It was so cold (about forty below zero) that I developed frostbite and I was almost screaming from pain when we reached his warm home and I started to thaw out. Everyone was in bed, and I started to dance around his bedroom trying to normalize my circulation. He was older than I, but a real farm boy and, although he tried to help me, thought the incident was pretty funny. It was a bloody awful experience, me dancing around the room trying frantically to alleviate the pain. I am sure it was funny—but not for me at the time.

The following morning, I met his wonderful family. After breakfast, I expressed my appreciation for their hospitality, and Russell took me to my grand-parents. To make the trip more comfortable, the family placed a couple of hot bricks by my feet in the sleigh for warmth. As I hadn't met my air force uncle or his bride, I felt so sorry for Russell's jilted sister, who was extremely attractive and loved my uncle. I was impressed that she and Russell had been so nice to me. I met them both at country dances thereafter, and they treated me as a family friend. Those country folk were wonderful and very pioneering in spirit and in giving of themselves.

Needless to say, without having received warning, my grandparents were sur-prised to have this very tall, skinny kid arrive at their doorstep. I had known very little about them. My grandfather was incredibly handsome with thick curly black hair, dark brown piercing eyes, and good features. He had an Irish back-ground and could be described as a Black Irishman. These Irish people originated during the time of the Spanish Armada in the late 1500s, when the Spaniards arrived in Ireland and propagated. My mother's family and virtually all of their offspring were blessed with my grandfather's good looks.

He had graduated from medical school in Toronto but decided to throw it all away to operate a well-drilling business. He ultimately combined this business with farming. He was very well read and extremely interesting. My father said he could look at a spread of land and smell the water table—it was that instinctive to him. I enjoyed lengthy conversations with my grandfather, who had a command-ing delivery as he told me stories regarding his family and the Munro family.

He admired my Munro grandfather tremendously for the management of his farmlands and his good business acumen in negotiating for cattle and other stock. My grandfather further stated that my Munro grandfather had been very prosper-ous and always negotiated every transaction fairly and honorably. He said he had done a lot of well-drilling over the years at my Munro grandfather's seven square miles of farmland. He said my Munro grandfather had been a prominent and well-respected farmer and had been treated with deference in their community. My father somewhat grudgingly had made the same statements, but with a some-what negative connotation.

Apart from the Depression years, thought I on numerous occasions, *What the hell happened to us?*

My grandfather, great at reminiscing, mentioned that he and a son-in-law were once trying to lift an oversized tool cabinet onto a wagon. He and the son-in-law were both very strong, but couldn't lift it. My grandfather suddenly saw my father coming toward them and he informed the son-in-law that he was about to solve the problem. As my father approached them, my grandfather casually asked my father to load the tool cabinet onto the wagon. Without further ado, my father simply picked it up and put it on the wagon. The son-in-law was a Scottish immigrant and became my father's best friend. My father had figured out what they were up to with the tool cabinet, and he gave them a demonstration of his strength, then simply walked off. My modest father's brawn was widely discussed—by everyone but himself.

My grandmother was an absolute sweetheart and originally hailed from North Dakota. She was Austrian and definitely of peasant stock. She was immaculate with herself, her dress, and her home. Her farmhouse was spotless, despite the fact that they had no inside plumbing or electricity. You could eat off of her floors. She was a devout Catholic and loved her church and her family. During the winter she stayed close to home, as travel was confined to horse and sleigh. However, during the rest of the year she loved traveling by car with my grandfather to get to town and to visit family and friends in the surrounding community. She could be eagerly ready to leave at a moment's notice.

Her cooked and baked goods were out of this world and so effortlessly prepared. Ironically, she loved store bought bread as a treat. She referred to it as "baker's bread." I was in hog heaven with her homemade bread and freshly churned butter, and all of the other baked goodies. I particularly loved her baking powder biscuits, and my grandfather would join me in teasing her to make them. To continue the teasing, she would hold back from making them.

One day my grandfather was going to town and I stayed home with my grandmother. She had been after him to clean the chicken pen. It was early spring and the pen really needed a good cleaning. To surprise them both, as soon as my grandfather left for town, I went out and spent the day cleaning the chicken pen. Late in the afternoon and before my grandfather arrived home, my grandmother called me into the kitchen. She had made me a tray of her delicious biscuits. I sat down and ate them all! We laughed and decided to keep it a secret. The joys of hog heaven—oink, oink! My grandmother was such a sweetheart. She worked so diligently at homemaking and was such a good example to me that her wish was my command—I would do anything for her.

During the colder months, my grandfather and I would ride their two horses to a special location to water them. The first day, as we approached the barn I asked my grandfather for a saddle. He said I was no longer a city boy and I had to ride bareback. Unlike the rest of my family and relatives, I did not care for horses—or to ride them. My parents were both great horse people, but not I.

Northern Manitoba is blessed with many lakes and very heavily wooded forests. Even in the farmlands, there were expanded areas that remained untouched forest and bush country. My grandfather, who was originally from Ontario, spent many years farming and drilled wells in southern Saskatchewan, which was sparsely treed. He had absolutely no trees on his small farm of eighty acres. Aside from a kitchen garden and some acreage to grow hay for their two horses and a cow, the rest of the land was devoted to barley.

His well-drilling business augmented his income. Because of the openness of his farm, the winds and dry, blowing snow would remind one of a desert. The snow was like the sand. When returning from the watering well the first time, my horse actually got down and started to roll in the snow. Fortunately, my grandfather was watching closely and yelled for me to get out of the way. After that experience, I decided to develop a better rapport with my horse rather than repeat the incident. My grandparents quickly realized I was no cowboy.

From where they lived we had a magnificent view of the northern lights as they danced across the sky in the evenings. It was a spectacular sight to behold, and unbelievably exciting to witness. Coming from a metropolitan background, I surprisingly enjoyed the quietude of a rural setting.

My mother must have learned from my sister Laura that I had left Vancouver and that I was visiting relatives until late spring, and thereafter rejoining my sister and her mate.

My mother took this opportunity to vindictively correspond with her family members. She included prevaricating innuendoes about my father with regards to my leaving home. I immediately perceived that my grandparents and other family members were extremely discreet in asking about both of my parents. They kept their inquires on a superficial level, which I appreciated. It would have been untenable of me to make disparaging remarks about either parent. My relationships with my relatives, to this point, were flowing beautifully and I was enjoying being with "kinfolk" whom I had never previously met. It seemed to enhance my personal perception of myself and, frankly, gave me a greater dimensional feeling of belonging.

One of my aunts lived nearby, and I remembered my father telling me that she was his favorite sibling in my mother's family. Unfortunately, she and her husband lost their first three children in a house fire. My aunt, leaving the children alone for a very brief period of time, went to the next farm to borrow something. The children were in bed, and just after my aunt left, one of the pipes came loose on their potbellied stove, sending the home instantaneously up in smoke. Sadly, the children expired from smoke inhalation.

Fortunately, the couple started a new family and had three more children when we met. Because of her horrible, tragic experience, my aunt had become a very precautious parent. She was really grateful for me to spend time with their children, and I enjoyed babysitting with them. On my first babysitting assignment she suggested that we negotiate a fee for my services.

In those days, all farms had root cellars—either within the home or adjacent to it—where they stored their larder. It was a natural place for storing fruits and vegetables. I checked their root cellar, came back with a quart of preserved peaches, and laughingly said, "This is my fee." My aunt responded with laughter and it became a joke between the two of us, as that was my remuneration each time. By the time she returned home the quart jar was always empty. And all consumed by me, the skinny babysitter. (Apart from a workplace, I would never ever charge anyone for babysitting or performing other chores. I always volunteered just to be helpful.)

Before early spring, it was decided that I would spend several weeks with an aunt and uncle—a young couple with five little children. They lived about twenty miles or more away and they had recently acquired a farm. The aunt was my mother's sister, and both she and my uncle were great people. My uncle had actually logged trees on his farmland and transported them to a small sawmill that transformed them into lumber to build their home.

During my stay with them, my uncle and I cleared forty acres of land to add to their barley crop acreage. He was multi-talented in the transformation of farmland and the ongoing construction of their home and other buildings for stock and storage. We worked long hours and I truly enjoyed farm life and looked forward to mealtimes, my remuneration, as my aunt was a great cook. She'd had a great teacher—my grandmother—and my aunt even resembled my grandmother in appearance.

My uncle loved my sense of humor and I would mimic one of the local farmers and his brother, who were both blessed with more than a few idiosyncrasies.

The brother of the farmer could not speak; he just simply muttered incoherently, and we were never certain of his level of comprehension, although he worked very adeptly and industriously. On one occasion, I was doing some work at my uncle's brother's farm that was adjacent to my uncle's farm. We were breaking new land for cultivation.

To begin with, after scrubbing the land of bush and trees, we had to remove the remaining tree stumps and rocks with a breaking plow, which was attached to a tractor. My job was to stand on a plank attached to the breaking plow to weigh it to the ground as the farmer drove the tractor. Each time we came to a large rock or heavy stump I would invariably fall—ass over teakettle as they used to say—in the process. I was slightly over six foot one, but weighed only about one hundred and forty pounds. When my uncle's brother had to leave for a few minutes, I decided to be a prankster.

The neighboring farmer's mute brother was helping us, and I persuaded and coached him on how to operate the tractor. The field was loaded with tree stumps and rocks, and he soon realized that he was over his head in trying to maneuver the tractor among all of the debris. He was in a frightful panic and he was waving his hands and arms wanting me to intercede and get him off the tractor. Instead, I was on my knees in hysterical laughter watching his performance, and then seeing my uncle's brother, returning on foot at a run screaming at me to help the "driver."

Watching the two of them only made me laugh even more uncontrollably. Yes, I got in trouble, but when I told my uncle of my prankish act, his reaction was the same as mine. My uncle and I shared ambivalent feelings about his brother.

My uncle and I had become best buddies; he was unequivocally one of my favorite relatives. He was very quiet and quite reserved, but I truly admired his work ethic and his tenaciousness in getting his projects completed. Thinking back, I wish he had received some kudos from both sides of his family. He was kind of a Lone Ranger. He appeared reclusive by nature, but definitely did not behave that way with me.

I think he admired my ongoing voluntary willingness to freely support him, and, in the process, we became very close. He would freely discuss his thoughts on family members and he was interested in hearing about my father and my perception of my family and our relatives. He said he would really like to meet my father some day, I assume disbelieving some of the negative comments he had heard. He was always so agreeable in siding with me on my family assessments, and he loved my adolescent sense of humor. I was his helping hand and comedian. My aunt quietly informed me that I was one of the few persons my uncle felt so strongly about. That pleased me tremendously, as the feeling was mutual.

On several occasions, my uncle would mention that my air force uncle, who had just returned from service with a new French Canadian bride, was the apple of my grandfather's eye. Being a son-in-law, he always felt that he had been relegated to second class. I surmised he had hurtful feelings, rather than envy.

In his rehabilitation to private life, my air force uncle became a successful refrigeration engineer and opened and maintained several frozen food lockers in the Swan River district. He was a great person, too, and had a wonderful family. I have always admired industrious individuals, and both uncles had the same excellent traits and should have been buddies in the family; but, paradoxically, I don't believe a friendship ever materialized.

Aside from helping to clear land on his brother's farm, I continued to offer my services to help my uncle achieve his goals in developing his farmland. In appreciation, my uncle would hitch up his horse and buggy for me to visit my grandparents who lived about two hours away. I loved the countryside—the grain fields, forests, and small rivers. While I hated horseback riding, I loved traveling by horse and buggy. The horse hoof sounds were pleasing on deserted roads.

I actually loved farming. I could do the rough menial chores, but, coming from the city, I was pretty awkward—not too handy at carpentry or mechanical projects. Frankly, and with apologies, I couldn't fix shit—I was a real dud.

It was equivalent to a great sabbatical to spend those few months farming with my relatives and getting to know them and learning country living. On one occasion, I saw a Native Canadian leading a horse that was attached to a travois in which his wife was sitting. (A travois is an A-frame made of two poles, across which a seating or cargo platform is attached. Such frames were pulled by man, dog, or horse since prehistoric times.) This was 1946, nearly a year after the end of World War II, and their method of transportation seemed so primitive to me. It was unbelievable to experience such a scene—reminiscent of the old West.

One early morning while I was staying with my aunt and uncle, I noticed a large creature crossing our main field. It was so huge I believed it to be a bear. However, about an hour or so later, a posse of neighborhood farmers, complete with shotguns, came by to inquire if we had seen the large timber wolf they were hunting. I believe the search party did track him down that morning. In the woods and bush lands of my uncle's farm there were many deer roaming around. On any given day we would see two or three deer romping through my uncle's forest reserve lands.

Frankly, I felt a little sad and nostalgic having to say farewell to my extended family. I had grown to love and admire them so quickly. In being with them, I had never experienced a moment of uncivil discourse, and I felt part of each family. But, I had carefully maintained my independence.

My Aunt Jessie, wife of the clergyman, and my father's sister, was very special to me. She was certainly a Munro, and she and my father strongly resembled one another in facial features. She dressed tastefully and had a commanding demeanor. She was extremely bright, spoke quietly and articulately, and was akin to my father in terms of being inherently an outstanding and thought-provoking conversationalist. They both spoke so quickly and they both conversed with me in engaging adult terms.

When my uncle was out of town attending church conferences and conducting church business, my aunt often conducted their church service. Her son Munro quoted me the following, "When my mother preaches the sermon, she doesn't rely on notes. The church congregation believes she is a remarkably talented lady to simply conduct off-the-cuff sermons." My aunt modestly smiled when hearing his comments.

I absolutely adored my grandparents—the original odd couple. He was a brilliant and well-read man and spoke with me also in an adult manner. My grandmother appeared very plain and simple, but was an incredible lady—so talented in cooking, sewing, and all of the great domestic pursuits that women of her generation excelled in. She was very witty and we had great fun together. She told me that she would stop by my bedroom while I was sleeping just to look at me. She remarked, "When you're asleep, you look like an angel, and when you're awake, you are such a mischievous brat!" When we were alone and in a playful mood, she would point out some of my grandfather's idiosyncrasies—nothing disparaging, just comical stuff. And we would laugh and laugh. When he displayed these traits in person, my grandmother and I would wink or nod to one another smilingly. I loved them both.

I adored my quiet uncle who was married to my mother's sister. He was my best audience for my own humor among my relatives. And he would laugh full heartily at my mimicry, while shaking his head at my antics. There was never an utterance of personal feelings, but he and I, while out in the field or bush working our butts off, would suddenly stop, look at each other and laugh thunderously over nothing. I believe it was our sign of affection and mutual admiration. We simply enjoyed the fun of having a good friendship and getting his projects fulfilled. He was so handy—a mister fix-it. He was a doer and a tremendous role model for me. He was so self-motivated and he used his great pioneering spirit to achieve the fulfillment of his dreams. When not working, he was totally devoted to his wonderful wife and children—no wild parties or poker games for that structured and disciplined young man. And he was an inspiration to me and definitely my favorite uncle, even though he was an uncle through marriage and we did not share a bloodline.

7

As summer approached, I said farewell to my farming relatives and rejoined my sister and her boyfriend. I met up with them in a farming town in southern Manitoba. My sister's first comment to me was, "Let me see your teeth. You have not been brushing them three times a day. As of today, no excuses, do you hear me?"

"Yes! I have been a farm boy—out at the crack of dawn and returning early evening." (I failed to mention that we had our main meal at noontime.)

Laura's mate was really glad to see me. He started teasing me immediately.

As we had planned, after a speedy orientation from my sister and her mate, I operated the popcorn concession that he jointly owned with another person. I worked like a robot; however, I did enjoy meeting people and they were kind and friendly. I loved traveling from town to town.

I was the youngest person working on any of the concessions. My daily receipts exceeded those of many other concessions, and, on one rainy location, exceeded them all. The owner and his wife heard laudatory comments about my daily performance. They informed my sister and mate that they would like to set up a new food concession for the next year that would be operated by me along with the owner's son. My sister and mate beamed with pride at me when I was singled out by the owner. However, I was cool on the idea, realizing that the carnival life was a youthful adventure and I might not want it to become a lifestyle. During the planning stages, I quietly and discreetly remained noncommittal. I thought, *Just let it ride.*

I slept in a big tent where my sister's mate, during show time, performed his act. I never saw the mate's performance—I was too busy being a popcorn robot. I heard it was actually quite good. Also joining me at bedtime in the tent was a menagerie of the mate's costars, consisting of a badger, a silver fox, four chattering monkeys, and various reptiles—securely boxed. My bed was a mattress placed on top of the reptile box, if one could imagine that! My evening prayers included a plea for my circumstantial safety. My God, what a combination of wildlife campers—that included this skinny runaway kid. For some strange reason, I simply viewed this entire setting as a very adventurous experience and never gave it a second thought. Just imagine me sleeping on a box filled with poisonous rattlesnakes and Texas bull snakes—never mind waking up in the early morning to a silver fox licking my feet! At least it wasn't the badger—he was really mean. Occasionally, it would rain overnight, and the pattering of the rain on the canvas created a very warm and cozy atmosphere. By contrast, this scenario was certainly a far cry and diversion from the poker and party gang.

The mate's popcorn stand partner was from Eastern Europe and he operated a portable photo unit. The equipment was so primitive that he could only take mini headshot pictures with just of one or two persons only in each shot. Frankly, his feature attraction was himself. He was an immigrant who struggled with English; however, in the process he was an absolute riot. His language and his gestures made his efforts to draw in a crowd quite hilarious.

If three young ladies were approaching his unit, they would be greeted, as follows: "Hello, charming. Hello, beauty. And hello, glad! Here we are, and are we here? Let's get our photos taken—one by one or two together. It will make you very happy!"

Laura was a great mimic and she and the owner's wife were good friends. The photographer always had his unit stationed next to mine among the other concessions. The owner's wife, after hearing Laura's mimicry of him, stopped by to see me and to overhear the photographer soliciting customers. When she witnessed his shtick in person, she almost convulsed, she thought it was so funny. Despite his English language problems, he was very entrepreneurial in drumming up business for his photo-unit. Actually, screwing up the English language made him more colorful and created personal interest. The photographer was extremely opinionated, but realized I worked like a robot and brought in the money simultaneously. He appreciated my work and was kind to me.

Planning ahead, I had saved enough money for my return train trip home to Vancouver. I even had enough to go sightseeing in Winnipeg for a couple of days before my departure, staying at a moderately priced hotel. For some reason I loved that city. My traveling train companions were those four monkeys and the badger, who, at our destination were, by predetermination, to be given to the famous Stanley Park Zoo in Vancouver.

While we had been touring with the carnival, my sister and her mate informed me that I should take out my daily expenses from my cash drawer and a little extra for savings. In those days you could open a Postal Service savings account, and deposit any extra money, even in a small town. I realized that their partner the photographer was to receive half of the daily proceeds. Another portion went to the owner of the road show. I flatly refused to take a dime from my cash drawer, as I knew it was wrong. I considered such an act to be classified as thievery.

Long after I had left the road show, Laura's mate was still chastising me for not tipping the till. He told me I was a damn fool. Although I was somewhat naive, I had long since realized that the mate's value system differed from mine. While reading the announcements at church each week as a youngster, I often forgot them. But I did remember, "Thou shalt not steal."

In early fall, I returned to Vancouver to reluctantly rejoin the poker and party gang. My father was delighted to see me home again and we recounted my experiences and thoughts on our relatives, farming, and the road show. Through my father, I started working in a nearby sawmill. I was working on a conveyor belt and my duties were both laborious and boring. I would play mind games on geography, countries (size and population), vocabulary, and spelling. Being uneducated, my only solace, sadly, was that I had little to remember or forget. I had no vocational dreams and I didn't even seem to have any vocational attributes or proclivities. Educationally, I was in no-man's-land—with suppressive thoughts.

My father quietly blamed me for my defiance in leaving school and for leaving home to stay with relatives. He was absolutely clueless about my basic needs, and he was totally unaware of the anger I sheltered toward him based on his hedonistic lifestyle. That hideous pen incident still remained a painful memory.

One weekend, Cecil came for a visit and I took him to Stanley Park to see "my" monkeys. When we arrived at the zoo the monkeys appeared to recognize me. They say that absence makes the heart grow fonder, but I wasn't sure that held for me and the monkeys. As we were standing there, a couple of teenage boys started to tease them. Cecil bellowed out predictably, "Stop teasing them!"

One lad sarcastically asked, "Are those your monkeys?'

Pointing to me, Cecil replied, "No, they belong to him and his family!"

The lad, taken off-guard, apologetically said to me, "I'm really sorry!"

To mitigate the situation, and because there were others viewing the monkeys at the same time, I quickly introduced the four monkeys to the crowd, pointing out and naming each of them. Additionally, I informed them that, while bringing them to Vancouver by train, I had to run from the Banff train station to a store for food to sustain their needs until we reached Vancouver. I had been thankful that an alert and concerned trainman had made sure I arrived back just in time before the train pulled out. I said, "The monkeys and I have one thing in common—I don't like them and they don't like me." I pleased the crowd and we had a little question-and-answer session thereafter to complete my extemporaneous comments.

Cecil and I laughed later as he said, "Just like the old days."

"Yeah, me bailing you out—as usual."

A few weeks later, Cecil came for the weekend. And his mission was telling. "Gus, I have something to tell you and you may not be too happy."

"Cecil, what have you done now?"

"I am leaving Vancouver in two weeks."

"What!"

"I have decided that there would be more opportunities in Toronto."

"I cannot believe what I am hearing. You have a good job, why leave?"

"I want a new start a new life and I have definitely decided to move to Toronto. I want to get established and eventually meet someone nice and get married and settle down. That is my goal, Gus."

"I assume your Munro family is the last to learn of your plans?"

"Yes. I knew that you were going to be the tough one to have to tell. Maybe, down the road, you'll join me in Toronto?"

"Could be." said I, sad and distraught.

That weekend visit was somber, with none of our usual fun and games. I was shocked—thunderstruck—but there was nothing I could do. Cecil had decided to leave and that was it. He was not impulsive by nature, and I assumed he had thought it over carefully. I hopefully rationalized the situation by thinking that he would go back to eastern Canada, stay for a while, get homesick, and return to Vancouver.

At one of our parties, a young man who was a student at the University of British Columbia (UBC) came with a group from father's pub club. George was in his early to mid-twenties and majored in theological studies at UBC. Aside from that, he was president of the largest teen town center in Vancouver and extremely active in both civic and academic pursuits. I was seventeen and very interested in conversing with him because of his background and, particularly, as he was attending the university. After we became friends, he said he thought I was bright and he was perplexed as to why I was in limbo working in a sawmill—obviously lacking the pursuit of educational goals and any future direction. George spoke to me like a Dutch uncle and said that I needed to get back to school. He suggested courses in typing and accounting—some basic skills. He also implied that I needed to simultaneously strengthen my vocational background.

He suggested I seek a white-collar job that would offer advancement or open other doors of opportunity for me and complement my business courses.

His interest and encouragement touched me profoundly, as no one in our large circle of friends and acquaintances had demonstrated such interest. I had simply been a fly on the wall. Here was someone trying to open a new door for me.

I challenged his suggestions by critically pointed out what a failure I had been up to this point. I was a school dropout doing manual labor at a sawmill conveyer belt performing menial robotic tasks. And, excluding my sojourn to the Prairie Provinces and western Ontario, my only work had been as a hotel busboy.

He responded that circumstances rather than ability and potential had driven my life, and that definitely hit a cord with me. He assertively stated that I had above-average intelligence, and, in plain English, said, "Knock off the bullshit and to get your ass moving in the right direction!" Reinforcing his point, he stated that he wouldn't have discussed the subject if he had not been certain of his observations. Frank and straightforward individuals were my cup of tea, so he and I got along very well.

Inspired by my new friend George's pep talk, I immediately enrolled at Commercial High School taking evening typing and accounting classes as he had suggested.

Furthermore, I applied for a position at the T. Eaton Company, a large national department store chain. I started in the stockroom of the electrical department—a foot in the door, so to speak. I quickly learned the ropes in retailing and moved from the stockroom onto the sales floor. I also became involved in the display units.

The public bought virtually everything from the department store, which was the retail hub of the city. The store stocked linens, clothing, complete home furnishings, major and small appliances, lamps, hardware, wallpaper and paints, sporting goods, stationery and supplies, watches and jewelry—you name it. In Canada, all of the leading department stores also had full-service grocery departments on their lower levels and they offered specialty and gourmet items on their mezzanine floors.

The manager I reported to was about seven years my senior, and very polished and dynamic. He became very supportive of me and was aware of my limited educational background. He was extremely complimentary regarding my performance, recognizing that I took the initiative to learn new functions and to accept responsibilities in monitoring our merchandise for restocking and audit verifications.

While I worked at the store, I had taken a class in merchandising, and my manager even afforded me the opportunity to try to write newspaper advertisements for our department. He had a couple of other lads who worked part-time fulfilling similar duties to mine; one was the son of one of our prominent store managers. Frequently, my manager would admonish them for unsatisfactory performance and use me as a standard. While he was generously complimentary to me, I felt uncomfortable, although the other lads never fired any resentment in my direction; we actually got along well.

One of the key persons to my manager was a man near fifty, whom I believe had been unfairly demoted when the T. Eaton Company took over the David Spencer Department Store. He, too, was terrific to work with, and I learned a lot about retailing from him.

The lamp department was part of the electrical department, and was supervised by a wonderful lady. Periodically, she and I would have to go to the warehouse and perform audits of our stocked merchandise. This woman had been with Eaton's for many years and had come to Vancouver when Eaton's acquired Spencer's. She was very diligent and a no-nonsense person. She was originally from Newfoundland, which had recently been transformed from the first British colony to Canada's tenth province.

She was great fun and blessed with a wonderful sense of humor. She loved my singing voice and, while working diligently in the warehouse, she made me serenade her as we performed our laborious stock audits. Coincidentally, our manager had a great baritone voice and, while at the warehouse, he too would try to impress her with his voice. She would whisper smilingly to me that my voice was better than his. But it wasn't. She was either being overly kind or she was tone-deaf.

Those three persons I worked with at Eaton's were among the finest people I have ever known. They were so wonderful to me, and they treated me as a little brother and often invited me to their homes. I was the kid, but we all teased each other and worked hard and had fun in the process. I have very fond memories of working with those folks. I tried emulating their excellent retailing traits; however, I knew this field would never work into a career for me.

My department manager invited me to a Christmas party in one of the old fashionable apartment buildings in Vancouver where his in-laws resided. Coincidentally, at the party I was reacquainted with the alderman and his wife, whom I had met at camp years before. The party was in full swing and the alderman seemed somewhat "crocked"—he was hugging all of the women while his wife, who also appeared slightly inebriated, was up on the coffee table doing the Charleston and singing, "Yes Sir, That's My Baby." I was shocked and disappointed at their behavior at that party, as it was contrary to their behavior at our earlier meeting, but my sense of humor eventually prevailed.

One summer, one of the store executives had his son spend some time with us in our department. He was assigned to work with me. He was overwhelmed on busy sale days and amazed that I had all of our ducks in order—all of our sale items were available and moved very quickly. He was forever telling everyone how efficient I was under pressure. He stayed close to me on those hectic sale days and relied heavily on my expertise. On one sale day, another store executive, a friend of his father who also knew the lad, stopped by the department to purchase a toaster from him. When the lad showed me the sales slip I empathetically stated, "Your writing is illegible. This is embarrassing! He is one of our top executives!"

Said the lad, "I suggested he complete the sales slip; it's his writing not mine, Gus."

Nepotism!

One evening, my sister Marjorie, at age fifteen, was to appear in a school concert. She was part of a western dance group. While she was performing in the number, I suddenly had a very strange feeling about her welfare—nothing specific, just a gut feeling. I couldn't shake that thought the entire evening, although there was no visible indication to explain why I was experiencing this premonition. After that evening, she very suddenly and rapidly lost a tremendous amount of weight, and she had been fairly slim to begin with.

Upon examination, she was diagnosed tuberculosis and was immediately hospitalized in the specialized tuberculosis unit of the Vancouver General Hospital.

She, herself, accepted her condition matter-of-factly. She adjusted to the feasibility of a prolonged hospital stay by just taking one day at a time. My father was absolutely devastated about her condition and her lengthy confinement. During this period, he and I moved to a smaller apartment. Although working full-time, he would drown his sorrow over Marjorie's illness by hitting the bottle. It was another very difficult period. I worked at the department store, attended classes after hours, and managed to visit my sister at the hospital every single visiting day.

During that period I had been seeing my mother on an infrequent basis. My panicky father suggested that my mother be notified of Marjorie's illness, and that my mother be given immediate visitation rights. Marjorie had had no contact with my mother. Although Marjorie was an extremely outgoing person, we had to do some coaxing before she reluctantly gave my mother the green light to visit her. My mother came each week to the hospital to see her and was pleased to be somewhat reunited with us. However, unbeknownst to my mother, the relationship was only superficial from my sister's standpoint. Additionally, my mother requested to meet with my father some early evening following our first hospital visit.

She came to our apartment on three or four occasions and enjoyed talking with my father after those many years. They reminisced about their families, relatives, and old mutual friends. Politeness prevailed during each visit, and the atmosphere was unquestionably congenial.

Marjorie had her schoolwork sent by correspondence and really adjusted to being confined to the hospital for fifteen months. She did have lung surgery. The removal of the smallest lower lobe on the right side was followed by a procedure involving the phrenic nerve to pull up the diaphragm. Before her discharge, my father and I moved to a larger apartment, and the Provincial Health Services representative came to our home to inspect and approve our living accommodations. Marjorie had an excellent recovery because she adhered to the program prescribed by her doctors.

At evening classes, I had a wonderful typing teacher. One evening before the class started I asked her, "What are the prerequisites for being successful in business?" (I did not, of course, mention my limited and dismal educational background.)

Her reply was both spontaneous and, momentarily, very profound. She said, "Business is simply a matter of keeping up with the times."

When I encouraged her to elaborate, she said, "I have known several businessmen who had limited formal education but who were very successful in the management and operation of their respective organizations. They simply applied my first comment."

Her comments were encouraging, but I was skeptical, thinking they were, perhaps, an oversimplification.

After completing my high school evening business introduction classes, I enrolled in a business college. The department store was closed each Wednesday, enabling me to attend classes all that day, and I also attended two evening classes each week. After I had attended classes for several weeks, one of my teachers pulled me aside and surreptitiously suggested I leave and enroll in a certified matriculation college to qualify to write university entrance examinations. I felt flattered as I realized that she had confidentially singled me out. She made laudatory comments in terms of my potential. I accepted her comments as music to my ears momentarily, until self-effacement resurfaced its ugly head. And that was to become an ongoing pattern for me in my struggling years.

I truly believe my sense of humor helped me tremendously in getting through those difficult periods during my youth—along with my boundless energy. Based on my former teacher's recommendation, I enrolled at the matriculation school and my first subject was algebra. I actually started with a private tutor. She started me off reviewing all basic arithmetic, which struck my sensitive nature as being somewhat demeaning. But, during my fifth session with her, she informed me that I had surpassed the full-day students, who had been in class each day for two months.

I thoughtfully, as a complete uninformed novice, examined the prerequisites for obtaining my university entrance. Based on my very limited viewpoint, I believed that none of the subjects would be beneficial to me in advancing in the business world per se. I was required to take a course in French and other classes that I believed would not enhance or strengthen my skills in working in a business office environment.

To begin with, I had no direction or desire to pursue a specific vocation or profession that required a set of prescribed educational standards. Therefore, I left the matriculation school to try to pursue other career opportunities; however, I lacked both foresight and direction.

While I was working at the T. Eaton Company, one of the assistant managers in another department was very impressed with my conscientious performance at the store. Her husband was a CPA who had acquired his own accounting firm. She convinced him to accept me in his accounting firm by offering an apprenticeship with the proviso that I continue taking intermediate and advanced accounting. Unbeknownst to me, they had fulfilled all of the preparatory work.

I thought at the time, *He must have had great respect for his wife's assessment to make such an offer.* The apprenticeship would help to strengthen and enhance my background with on-the-job experience along with continuing education. It was a wonderful opportunity, which I had to reluctantly turn down, as I realized in just studying basic accounting principles that accounting was also not my forte. I did treasure her kindness and confidence in recognizing my work attributes enough to provide this generous offer. I had been at the store for over two years and realized I would never contemplate or pursue a career in either retailing or accounting.

At that time, one of my colleagues at work had also been taking business classes and he mentioned that the Canadian Pacific Railway Telegraph Office had some open clerical positions. My typing skills were still somewhat marginal; however, I decided to apply for a position and was accepted.

The T. Eaton Company was blessed in having John Earle, an efficacious man under forty years old, in one of their leadership positions. He was the epitome of a topnotch executive. At my farewell gathering, we were all shocked that he had usurped my manager by surprisingly calling all departments under his personal direction and inviting them to gather and witness my farewell sendoff.

My duties had been so menial compared to his. I was amazed that he totally understood the basic functions that I had performed. It seems he had witnessed me in the process of diligently completing my assignments.

He said to the group that my dedication and loyalty to the organization was absolutely commendable. Furthermore, I would have had an excellent future had I remained with their company. Those compelling words rang in my ears and I felt joyful.

After his glowing and praiseworthy comments, the only one more spellbound and shockingly impressed than myself was my upstaged but grateful manager. "Gus, what a compliment to you; I have never witnessed such a complimentary speech from John Earle."

I had worked so hard at home and had never received one sign of appreciation from my father or any other member of my family. Needless to say, this grade-school dropout, riddled with the constant fear of failure, had never received such praise. However, I believe my manager was even more overwhelmed with appreciation than I was. That was another compliment to me, as he had been so encouraging and kind to me from the day I had started working in his department. He also greatly admired John Earle, which completed the picture of my departure with fulfillment.

8

I started at the Canadian Pacific Telegraph Office in their service department. That department addressed the needs of customers and also was actively involved in the actual railway communication services. I worked in that department for a few months and then transferred to the message center as an operator. This department accepted incoming telegrams from businesses and individuals. We also received overseas cables, press communications, and incoming messages from other telegraphic offices, both domestic and from other countries.

We used manual typewriters; however, they were specially modified to include upper case only for faster typing. My typing and spelling skills were both challenged, along with my communication and public relation skills, while I worked in that department.

In the early 1950s, teletype equipment typists and Morse code operators were responsible to cover virtually all communication needs, apart from the telephone, radio, postal, and delivery services. The telegraph offices were essential to business, industry, and personal communications. Teletype equipment was installed in large-volume organizations and used internally and in networks with their other offices or plants, and used externally with direct services to and from the telegraph offices.

I worked in the main office in Vancouver; there were several smaller branch offices throughout the city. I had worked a few months in the communications department when someone in management approached me to apply for the position of relieving supervisor. I was appreciative of being singled out by management for this position; however, I responded that I had not been in the job long enough to achieve seniority. Management countered my response by stating that they could use the "ability clause" in addressing any stipulation with the union.

Surprisingly, I became utility supervisor, relieving the day supervisor on the weekends, and the night supervisor on Monday and Tuesday nights. I worked as an operator on Wednesdays. I was twenty-one and we had a staff of twenty persons covering both shifts, aged from nineteen to sixty-four. In deference and with perfect promotional timing, I sent the lady who was sixty-four a valentine and she gratefully blushed. And she supported me strongly.

In my department and other departments, there were a lot of young people, both girls and guys, in the organization and we did a lot of social activities together. Many of us worked evenings and weekends and our inflexible work schedules drew us more closely together. We attended movies, parties, dances, dinners and other social events. We also went to the beaches and we had a lot of fun. At one time, we had the cousins of both the actress Arlene Dahl and actor Glen Ford working in our department. We were somewhat unsophisticated, provincial, and star struck.

On one occasion, two work colleagues and I were having a few beers after hours. Before leaving the premises, I decided that each one of us should put a glass of beer in each of our two overcoat pockets and take them to my staff at work. I must add that the hotel beer parlor was conveniently just behind our office—a stone's throw away. We stopped by and, as true Canadian colleagues, they apparently loved my gesture and the cold beer. However, when they were finished, being prankish, the staff decided to leave the empty glasses in my locker. The following day, I went to get my headset from my locker before my meeting with the day supervisor for shift instructions. When I opened my locker, all of the empty beer glasses tumbled out in her presence—one of my more shocking, totally off-guard experiences. However, I promptly and ambidextrously took care of the situation while quickly engaging in conversation with her regarding any instructions for the evening that needed to be addressed. I received no comment from her, but I definitely learned a lesson—no more beer.

Before I started in the communications department, I would assist the delivery department along with performing my duties in the service unit. The delivery department manager was an older man, who wore his glasses halfway down his nose and peered at people in a very strict manner—sternly but not condescendingly. He could admonish an employee without batting a piercing eye.

One day, I made a minor error, but was very uncomfortable in bringing it to his attention. He, unlike all of the staff, called me "Angus" rather than "Gus." I thought it quite interesting and it struck me as a personalizing gesture as I placed him internally in a VIP category. When I approached him somewhat awkwardly and apologized for my faux pas he brushed it aside saying, "When one works as hard as you do, one occasionally makes mistakes … nothing to worry about."

His nonchalant response really surprised me, as I had seen others severely and openly reprimanded on similar occasions. No one volunteered to mess with him under any circumstances, as he could be a hellion.

The (female) communications supervisor, whom I reported to at the time, met with this man on a regular basis. Being in a mischievous mood one day, I approached him and asked what was going on between himself and the communications supervisor. He looked at me rather strangely and said, "Angus, what are you talking about?"

I replied, "She has her eye on you. She is divorced and you are married." No one went beyond his sternly persona with such foolishness, and he loved it. When he was meeting with her in my presence, I would wink at him and he would start to laugh; he would confront me later,

"What are you trying to do by embarrassing me?"

We would laugh and I would say, "Well?" He realized that no one teased him, nor, in their right mind, conceived of him as a Casanova. He loved my humor and teasing. If this situation had backfired I would have been in serious trouble. He thought I was both industrious and a conscientious employee, but socially an outrageous and incorrigible brat.

To my credit, I am certain he realized that I was extremely confidential and did not share our lighter moments of teasing and comments with anyone else. He was truly from the old school, but we developed a great friendship; we had happy times working together. A little silliness among dedicated workers can be a very personally rewarding experience, once you open that door of opportunity.

One of my job priorities as relieving supervisor was to personally notify an addressee by telephone when we received messages of bereavement. Needless to say, this was an important daily function, but sadly unpleasant to address. I did my best in screening the calls to be certain I spoke with the appropriate persons. Each person responds differently to bad news, and there is one situation that I vividly recall. I called a lady and informed her of the following, "I am sorry to inform you that Joe passed away very suddenly this morning."

The distraught lady, bless her heart, responded by shouting to her husband, "Get off of your ass, Joe just died!" Poor guy what could he possibly do?

On a more pleasant note, the British Commonwealth Games were held in Vancouver in 1954. Dr. Roger Bannister had previously run the mile in less than four minutes. His actual time was 3 minutes, 59.4 seconds—and a record in track that year at Oxford. He called our office to send a cablegram to the United Kingdom. He had just defeated his leading competitor, John Landy, an Australian, in about a four-minute run. I had the pleasure of taking the message and speaking with him. These two incidents had been hot major events in the track world in 1954.

I believed that if my circumstances had been different, I would have enjoyed and done well participating seriously in track—or speed walking. My favorite cousin was the welterweight amateur boxing champion of Manitoba and personally had to do a lot of roadwork. When we were together in Vancouver or Flin Flon, Manitoba, he would say, whether we were walking or running, "Who can keep up with you?'

When I finally surpassed my father in speed walking, I said, "Hurry up, slowpoke, as my day has come."

One of the company solicitors would often join some of the members of our staff for a few beers after work. He was excellent at his position; however, he was married and had a reputation for running after the ladies. Coming from a broken home, I was somewhat intolerant of that lifestyle, knowing how it had greatly affected my life.

He was married and he was certainly no Romeo, but, over a few drinks, he would boringly discuss his escapades with the ladies. I made a mental note never ever to discuss my love affairs with anyone after listening to his monotonous commentary.

While I had negative feelings about him, he apparently paid me the best compliment I received while working at the railway. A colleague informed me that he was having a few beers one evening with the solicitor, who stated, "If our Montreal main office knew they had a twenty-two-year-old supervisor working successfully with a staffing complement ranging from under twenty to sixty-five years, they would promotionally send him back East."

During my conversation with my colleague, he went on to say that the solicitor was right. He said that, apart from working well with others, I possessed managerial qualities that he and other fellows in our group did not possess. While I was unsure of myself at the time, it did give me a boost and something to ponder over in terms of my future expectations. I also learned that you can receive commendations from unexpected sources.

I enrolled at what was then the Vancouver Vocational Institute (it is now Vancouver City College) located within walking distance from my office. My relieving supervisory position enabled me to attend day classes in the business school. The teacher conducting the programs befriended me and he and I would often have lunch together. He informed me that, while I was in the same age group as many of the students, he considered me an adult who worked independently and required minimal instruction and produced quality assignments.

The school aligned its faculty and educational programs to both industry and commerce, and they placed many of their graduate students directly to employers. On several occasions, when good positions were available, my instructor tried to send me on interviews. I occasionally went to appease him, but, frankly, I wanted to remain at my current position and continue classes. One day at class I overheard a conversation between two adult students; they were making praiseworthy comments about the merits of working for an oil company. They mentioned the companies by name and I made a mental note.

I met a very attractive young lady at work. Rose was the manager of one of our branch offices. Aside from her good looks and tasteful dress code, she had excellent typing and telegraphic machine skills. She was incredible. We immediately fell madly in love. The railway was unionized, and married couples could not be jointly employed. When we contemplated marriage, we decided on a quiet wedding. This enabled us to transition and work out new employment plans for both of us.

In Vancouver, employment opportunities were few. I clearly remembered the students' conversation regarding the benefits of working for an oil company.

I applied for a position with the British American Oil Company. I simply walked in off the street, and had three interviews that same day. I received a call at home that evening, informing me that I had a job in their credit department. On my first working day, a friendly Englishman sitting at the desk behind mine stated that I had been selected over approximately one hundred other applicants. He and his wife had come to Canada from the United Kingdom with the expectation of moving to the United States after establishing a two-year Canadian residency.

Frankly, I knew nothing about credit management when I joined the company. In order to be hirable, it was stipulated that I must agree to enroll in a special program sponsored through the University of Toronto. Each department had specific occupational needs. The University of Toronto developed and tailored applicable programs to enhance employee skills and performance for our organization and many others. In my case, I attended a study program for three years, taking five courses each year and applying for approval by the Canadian Credit Managers Association. Upon completion of the study program, I was required to fulfill an apprenticeship of five years of practical experience in credit management before receiving my certificate. I considered this an enhancement program for me.

I started as an assistant to one of the regional senior credit men. He was responsible for a geographic section of British Columbia. We worked closely with our district agents in approving credit and managing their customer accounts.

Their customers represented a mix of large and small businesses—farmers, ranchers, miners, fishermen, and other individuals and groups that needed petroleum products. Aside from the district agent, we also worked closely with our district sales force, as they assisted the agents in maintaining and generating new business. We also worked directly and indirectly with our service stations and other outlets.

My senior, Jack, worked diligently on contract issues and other managerial services. I received the checks and billing correspondence and was responsible for following our assigned accounts to be certain that payments were received on time.

As I sat next to Jack, I would listen to him dictating correspondence. I also took note of the many speeches he made within the organization. He was chairperson of our employee committee and was actively involved in many business and employee issues. His writing and speaking skills were very courteous, clear, and concise, and he spoke with very ingratiating intonations. This experience was both a job and classroom for me.

I recall working my monthly follow-up of all of my accounts my second month at work. Upon reviewing the accounts, I realized that I should have taken more effective steps in my prior follow-up. Jack was a very affable guy. When I subtly mentioned to him that in reviewing my first follow-up, I had to confess that my decision-making had not been as effective as it should have been. Unexpectedly, he roared with laughter and patted my shoulder and exclaimed, "Great! You are very quickly learning the ropes!"

His simplistic communication style rubbed off on me. I realized the tremendous impact he had on both my writing and speaking skills—I apparently learned them from him by osmosis. We had a secretarial pool and a communication system in which we used a telephone that was wired directly into their unit. After nervously dictating my very first letter, I realized that one of my colleagues had been standing behind me, listening to me conveying my dictation. "Gus, I just overheard your letter. You mentioned options as a solution, which was great. I wanted to offer the same, but didn't know quite how to say it. Thanks for your indirect help." Nice compliment to receive on my very first dictated letter.

I worked with Jack for a few months and was promoted to the retail credit card section, where I worked for a short period of time. Thereafter, in less than two years from my first day of employment, I was promoted to a comparable position to the one Jack held. Jack was a strong supporter.

It was pointed out internally on several occasions that I had been the most quickly promoted person within the department—and actually the organization.

I worked in that position a year or so, but, because of a serious ongoing sinus condition, I moved to California, believing that a drier climate would be beneficial.

I also arranged to continue the program through the University of Toronto and the Canadian Credit Managers Association after my resettlement and with the guidance of a self-selected proctor in the West Los Angeles School District.

Before I left Vancouver, the general credit manager, a somewhat quiet and very conservatively thoughtful man, called me into his office with a word of advice. He stated that my performance had been outstanding with their organization and I would be welcomed back should the occasion arise. He further took the opportunity to state that I was too self-deprecating and judgmental and that I personally felt totally responsible for anything that took place within my area, regardless of the circumstances. He advised that, when complex or irritating issues occur, I should just stop for a minute and discuss them with one of my peers and try to lighten up. His observations were very astute. It took me years to realize just how poignantly profound his comments were. His surname was actually Wiseman—a perfect match.

A couple of my colleagues informed me that there would be a farewell party held for me. I was slightly concerned anticipating my last day. A few weeks prior, one of the other young men had left the company and a get-together had been held for him at a nearby hotel. Sadly, the colleague leaving, our general credit manager and his assistant, and I had been the only people who showed up. It was an incredibly embarrassing moment for us all. We made light of it and tried to make that colleague feel better by complimenting him for his good work.

When I arrived at my own farewell party, everyone was there and a wild evening was in store. The party continued for another three hours after my departure. I heard that they all returned to work on Monday looking sheepish for the craziness that had occurred after I had left. Apparently, a good time was had by all—until the hangovers hit. We Canadian beer-guzzling chaps were all so young and foolish.

I was twenty-six and soon to be twenty-seven. In numerology, the twenty-seventh year is a major milestone in one's life. I recapped my recent life, grateful for the suggestion of my UBC theological student friend, who had told me to get off my ass and get moving!

While working for the Canadian Pacific Railway Telegraph Company and British American Oil Company I had been recognized promotionally for fulfilling my duties in an effective manner. Those in the workplace—my biggest fans—had cheered me on.

Frankly, with my limited educational background, I found myself somewhat bewildered in realizing that I was able to function so proficiently. While employed with the T. Eaton Company, Canadian Pacific Railway Telegraph Company, and British American Oil Company I received many complimentary comments from management, peers, and customers regarding my effective performance. I had a tremendous amount of fun working with everyone. Unfortunately, my personal fears of inadequacy, whether they were realistic or unrealistic, were carved in concrete. In my own mind, I was still the unappreciated kid janitor at home and a school dropout. I was internally a very angry and resentful young man based on those years of turmoil that followed our departure from the Inglehart family.

Apart from the sadness of leaving Vancouver, family, friends, and colleagues, my bride and I had a feeling of excitement as the day approached when we were to leave for California. We moved there "sight unseen" and with great anticipation.

My English buddy (from British American Oil) and his wife, along with another couple, met us at the Union Pacific Railroad Station when we arrived in Los Angeles. My English friend had told the group, "Look for a guy wearing a white shirt and red tie." They quickly found us. It was the red tie.

9

September 22, 1957, was our arrival date in Los Angeles. We immediately started to search for employment. At that particular time, many newcomers to the city were seeking employment opportunities through employment agencies. The advertisements in the *Los Angeles Times* listed column after column of open positions at these agencies. However, rather than exploring opportunities through the agencies, I decided to focus directly and personally within the petroleum industry. As I had been with British American Oil Company in Canada, my first contact for employment was with Richfield Oil Corporation. My former employer had a credit card exchange agreement with them and also with the Union Oil Company.

The Richfield Oil Corporation main office was located in downtown Los Angeles. The Richfield Building dominated the skyline in the city center with its magnificent art deco facade. I was so impressed with this towering structure, I decided that I wanted to work for Richfield Oil—in that building. Upon entering the street level, visitors knew immediately that they were in a corporate office, as it gleamed with immaculate care. The beams, walls, and the marble floors sparkled from cleanliness, and the atmosphere seemed to reflect tasteful conservatism. We had been told, while touring and sightseeing with our English friends, that, due to the threat of earthquakes, no building in Los Angeles was to exceed its tallest building at that time, which was the City Hall.

Unfortunately, my ebullience to work in the downtown building was shattered when I learned that their regional office housed their business services. That office was located in the fast-growing Wilshire Boulevard business district a few miles west from the downtown area. Being an old movie buff, I was impressed to learn that their office was located on the next corner to the original famous Brown Derby Restaurant (the one shaped like the hat). The Ambassador Hotel was located across the street—which housed the renowned Coconut Grove. Both places were popularized and patronized by what we now characterize as the old Hollywood elite. Even being an ardent movie fan, my druthers were still for the downtown building, as I was captivated by that impressive structure.

I was somewhat nervous that first morning, knowing I had to get out and start looking for a job. I was a newcomer to Los Angeles; I had been at home in Van-

71

couver. Los Angeles seemed gigantic to this new transplant that was not too cosmopolitan. I was an immigrant walk-in seeking employment in a strange city, fearfully hoping for acceptance and wondering if I could meet their criteria should they have any open positions.

I was keenly aware that, after the Korean War, my contemporaries in California attended college and I was looking at stiffer job market competition in Los Angeles than I had in Vancouver. And in terms of writing credentials, I would have to submit a blank piece of paper. My only solace was my work background that could be favorably verified. My astuteness took all of these issues into consideration, but I was still a grade-school dropout.

Nervously and unannounced, I arrived at the regional office to make employment inquiries and was sent directly to the credit department. From there, I was ushered into the office of the regional credit manager, Harry Swisher. Sometime later, I was informed that this gentleman was a direct descendent of the founder of the Swisher Company, a long-established and prestigious national organization known for their bathroom fixtures.

Harry Swisher was a short, paunchy gentleman, immaculately dressed and well groomed who appeared to be in his early sixties. He greeted me in a somewhat condescending manner; however, after our brief amenities, I politely took the initiative, as I definitely wanted a position in his organization.

"Mr. Swisher, I have just arrived from Vancouver, Canada, where I worked for British American Oil. I left a senior position in their credit department. I am very familiar with your organization. I am applying for a position here, as we have an excellent exchange agreement between our two companies. Your downtown main office building is magnificent with its impressive art deco facade."

"Mr. Munro, I have a great staffing complement and my newer employees are graduate students from both USC and UCLA. I have no unfilled positions."

"Mr. Swisher, in coming to a new company, and particularly a new country, I would expect to start at a lower position where I could prove myself before being considered for future promotions."

"We have had an exchange agreement with British American Oil so I am very familiar with that organization."

"Mr. Swisher, I would be very appreciative if you could keep my application on file for future employment possibilities."

"Sorry, I have nothing open and I don't anticipate any changes in staffing in the foreseeable future."

He stood up with an outstretched hand as I ended the conversation by saying, "Mr. Swisher, thank you for your time."

After my interview with Mr. Swisher, I felt totally distraught and crestfallen by his demeanor. He had spoken laconically and with a tone of indifference. The fears that had accumulated prior to the interview came to the forefront; however, I was able to rationalize that I came with a good work background. I felt the door was slammed in my face and no future options available to me.

I believe that, in terms of my general appearance, dress, manners and speech, and by not being overly assertive, I had presented myself favorably. I was totally crushed by Mr. Swisher's indifference during our brief meeting. Additionally, before it was ever opened, I had to close the door on any aspirations of being affiliated with the gold-domed building.

With Richfield Oil Corporation permanently off of my list of possible employment opportunities, I proceeded to apply to the Union Oil Company, the other reciprocal company on my list. I located their downtown office and entered it looking for their employment office. In the hallway, I ran into a young executive who informed me that I was in the corporate office. In his friendly manner, he directed me to the regional office. He stated that it was within walking distance. He told me to see the regional credit manager whose office was on the third floor. He even walked to the front entrance while pointing directions.

I followed his instructions and met with the regional credit manager. Mr. Miller was an older man, nice in appearance, and immaculately dressed. He was extremely gracious and receptive, especially as I had just walked into his office off of the street. This gentleman's friendly manner appeared to be the antithesis of Harry Swisher.

"So, Mr. Munro, you are from Vancouver. That is a beautiful city. What brought you south?"

"I have a chronic sinus condition and the wet weather is not conducive. As you know, my former employer, British American Oil, has an exchange agreement with your company and I am seeking a position."

"At the moment, I have nothing to offer. However, I anticipate a possible change coming shortly."

"I would be grateful for any consideration."

His phone rang. "Excuse me, Mr. Munro, I want to take this call."

I heard, of course, only his side of the conversation. "Hello … yes, John, he is in my office now … John, I totally agree and I would like to find him a position as well. I am hoping to bring him on staff in a couple of weeks if we can work it out … John, you are right. He presents himself impressively and he appears to be a great candidate for our organization … Thanks for your call."

Mr. Miller then addressed me, "Mr. Munro, that was one of our executives in our home office—he directed you to me. He was very impressed by your appearance and demeanor and believes, as I do, that you would potentially be an asset once we get you onboard. I am hoping to work something out for you and I definitely will be in touch with you in two weeks. I'm certain you realize I cannot definitely commit myself at this time, but I shall do my best."

"You and the other gentleman at the corporate office have been so kind to me, and I really appreciate being considered for a position. I want you to know that I come with good references and I take my work assignments very seriously."

As I left his office, I was overwhelmed with appreciation for the kindness exhibited by both of those men.

I felt quite optimistic and certainly more confident because of their laudatory comments and interest—and most of all because of their politeness to a newcomer who was desperately seeking acceptance. However, my sensitive nature had not forgotten or forgiven the very laconic, indifferent, and infamous Harry Swisher. We Scorpios are so unforgiving and vindictive.

As I was leaving the Union Oil Company regional office, I noticed a Standard Oil of California office across the street on the next block. Standard Oil also had an office in Vancouver and, as a matter of fact, my British American Oil coworker Jack had a brother who worked in that Vancouver office. Additionally, they had offices throughout Canada, so I was familiar with their company. I went to their personnel department and, after two interviews, I was hired. The interview process at Standard Oil was with the assistant credit manager, who not condescendingly but cautiously led me to believe that he had a dynamic staff and was not certain I would be able to meet the stiff competition. He very candidly emphasized that their hiring preference was to seek candidates with college degrees. I informed him that I would be continuing my education and realized how essential it was in progressing within any organization.

My Canadian background was not an issue, as he had relatives who lived in Victoria and other parts of British Columbia. He was courteous to me, but I could not understand why he had actually hired me. I felt I was being treated subordinately, which had been something that I had never experienced. I felt that the assistant credit manager had reluctantly hired me just to quickly fill an open position. In my entire employment history it was the only position I accepted under what I suspected to be subordinate circumstances. However, he commendably still hired this non-college applicant.

At the end of two weeks, the regional credit manager at Union Oil, as promised, contacted me and offered me a position. As I had already started working for Standard Oil, I thanked him and informed him that I had accepted another position. Because of my favorable experience initially with Union Oil, I often wondered if I should have accepted their position. While I pondered it over very carefully, I decided to remain at Standard Oil and build up my work experience. One never knows.

Shortly after our arrival in California, my wife and I were strolling down Figueroa Street in Los Angeles one Saturday when we saw a compact car with a British Columbia license plate. Jokingly, we thought maybe it was someone we knew. Considering the vastness of Los Angeles, seeing someone we knew would be classified as a near miracle.

I lowered my head and attempted to inconspicuously glance into the vehicle—and to my surprise, there was the Canadian Pacific Railway agent, Mr. Hickey sitting there. "Oh, my gosh," he screamed, "If it isn't Rose and Gus Munro!" We were all shocked, and our meeting was like old home week as we were all so happy to see one another. He kept looking at us in utter amazement and appreciation that we had been reunited in this large, strange city.

When I worked at the Canadian Pacific Railway Telegraph office in Vancouver, Mr. Hickey had been the general agent for the province. Most of my administrative issues and concerns were directed to his assistant, Mr. Killeen. However, the agent was very cognizant of our individual performance, and both men had been very instrumental in identifying my performance and recommending me for the position of relieving supervisor. I had been very grateful to both of these men for affording me that promotion. Technically, when I worked on the weekends at the CPR I was in charge of the Vancouver office, their third largest office in Canada.

I am certain that my position and supervisory experience at the CPR was a contributory factor to my obtaining a position with the British American Oil Company and also my next position at Standard Oil of California. My supervisory position at CPR initially started the ball rolling for me. And, as I look back, I am eternally grateful to the agent and his assistant for the opportunities bestowed on me while I worked in that office. Because I had flexible hours, I was able to attend classes and to enhance my overall resume.

Shortly after I started to work at Standard Oil, my father passed away very suddenly and unexpectedly in Vancouver. His health had greatly deteriorated, as he was an asthmatic and had previously been subjected to coal dust, plus he had been a very heavy smoker. My wife and I flew back to Vancouver to see our family and make the necessary funeral arrangements.

Unfortunately, we made the necessary arrangements before the service announcement of my father's passing could be printed in the newspaper. However, word quickly spread among our many wonderful family friends, and the service was performed to a full house.

Because of the circumstances, we were unable to make arrangements to have all of the guests at the funeral join us thereafter; however, I did take the opportunity to speak with each person there after the service. So many people had come—old family friends that I had not seen for many years. I was so pleased that they had come on such short notice.

Many said that my father had visited with them recently, and said that he was planning to return to the interior of the province to try and improve his health. The good lord had other plans.

Our flight to Vancouver had been my first experience in an airplane, and, right after takeoff, I quickly developed a fear of flying. We returned to California via train.

After briefly reporting to one condescending line supervisor at Standard Oil, I reported to another who was very impressed with my knowledge and believed that I should have a great future there. I did express my negative concerns and he assured me that he would be very supportive. We developed a good rapport and I had great respect for his performance and knowledge that made it very easy for us to work together. Our conversations were always frank and we shared a good sense of humor on our staff, issues, and workflow. He stood out among the crowd for his work ethic, his trustworthiness, and his integrity.

Ours was a large office and there were several positions in the retail credit card division. I had left a much higher position at British American Oil and realized I had to start over again. The work came very easily to me and my only learning curve was in familiarizing myself with Los Angeles and Southern California.

Word soon spread among my co-workers that I had good dictation skills, and, bypassing their supervisors, several of my colleagues would surreptitiously give me their dictation. They would make telephone calls for me in exchange.

The secretaries were in a pool and they were delighted that I was expanding my dictation. They said they each looked forward to my work, as it was the best in the department. I kept them very busy and content. I also had to address those spelling differences, between American English and Canadian English.

Inwardly, my inferior feelings and insecurities as a grade-school dropout were most prevalent during my tenure at Standard Oil. In Canada, I had had to compete with both high school and college graduates. Arriving in California, all of my contemporaries were college graduates. A brilliant co-worker, who later became a good friend, had received his master's and was working on obtaining a law degree.

While I could rationalize my feelings of insecurity, my co-workers, not knowing my true background, were most complimentary. Many befriended me apart from work. They viewed me as being well versed in business procedures and without hesitancy would call upon me for assistance and guidance. There were about eighteen young men occupying just our section of the office.

One Friday afternoon, before we closed for the weekend, the atmosphere was light and somewhat jolly. One of the guys asked how to spell a word and someone yelled, "Ask Gus." I responded by spelling the word and telling the group that I had noticed in Los Angeles that words were not correctly enunciated properly, thus creating spelling problems.

In the group was a young man who had a degree in English. I had perceived him to be extremely bright with the potential of a great future elsewhere. He loved these types of conversations and he egged me on by saying, "Gus, give us an example of your comments."

"Well, in California, if I need my teeth checked I go to the "dentist," whereas you Californians go to the "dennis." You slur your *T*'s and fail to enunciate them properly."

One yelled, "Hey guys, Gus has a point."

Another yelled, "Send that Canuck back to Canada—get him to hell out of here." We all roared and the conversation opened up with other examples and funny comments. It was a late Friday afternoon, and we all got an energy rush, just as children get that last minute burst of energy before bedtime. (By the way, my assumption of the English major was correct. He became a literary agent in New York City. I love bright people.)

There was one young man, Bob from Kansas, newly married, who started in our department a few months after I did. He seemed to be kind of a "good old boy" type. There was a young man, Jim from Oklahoma, with whom I normally had lunch, and we always left the office to go elsewhere to eat. Bob started to join us daily.

Bob had an inquiring mind; however, he would often ask me a work question. I would answer and then he would state that Jim or someone else did things differently. This seemed to occur on a daily basis and it started to irk me. Why bother me if you respect the opinion of someone else? He strongly focused on my dictation skills and he would ask numerous questions without being challenging or questioning my response. While I liked him, I felt like wringing his neck. One day, out of the blue, he stopped by my desk and, as I had just completed a recording of dictation for the secretarial pool, he grabbed the tape and counted the number of letters. He said, "Great, I have finally caught up and surpassed you by two letters!"

I defiantly said, "What does that mean?"

"You instructed me to write my letters clearly, concisely, and courteously and my volume now matches yours!"

"Thanks for the compliment. When you ask me a question on other issues, I give you an answer and you challenge me with the comments of others. What does that mean?"

"It means that you are a damn good teacher and mentor to me, Gus."

"Touché!"

Needless to say, with his unexpected and glowing comments, he definitely remained in my inner circle at Standard Oil. Later, other important opportunities arose for him within the corporation. He was requested to take specific examinations for promotional considerations and he passed with flying colors, having the highest marks in the selection process. I was so proud of him, but not surprised by his brightness—it had always been evident to me. His avocation was piloting private smaller planes.

The credit manager's secretary could be described as a down-to-earth, Southern belle. Aside from her secretarial duties, she actively addressed customer needs and complaints. She began to call upon me to assist her in the resolution of complaints she received by letter, phone, and in person. Strong on customer relations, she pulled me aside one day and stated, "You are the best person in the department to help me and our customers." A twinkle came into her blue eyes. "Apart from being well groomed, courteous, and businesslike," she added, "you shine your shoes every day." Dryly she added, "You are the Lone Ranger on shoes." She freely expressed her praiseworthy comments about me to the management team and the secretarial staff. She really appreciated employees that took that extra step on behalf of the customer and therefore ultimately benefited the organization. She was a refined lady, full of fun, and good for my shattered ego.

My supervisor reported to the office manager, who was an older man diminutive in stature and frail, and meticulous in his dress and manner. He possessed exemplary work habits and was responsible for giving our annual reviews.

He and the Southern belle had been with Standard Oil for many years. They were both adamant in their approach in maintaining good standards. They were perfectionists and professed ongoing loyalty to the organization. They both seemed to identify similar qualities in me, and we three became fast friends at work. We teased one another and I adored them both. I was more in tune with them because of their maturity than I was with most of my other co-workers in terms of customer relations and decorum. We three always seemed to take that extra step in resolving customer issues in a manner that was favorable to the customer and the organization.

I spent almost three years at Standard Oil, but realized from the beginning that my future was elsewhere. At no time during my employment at Standard Oil did I consider remaining there indefinitely. It was a nice place to work: I enjoyed the people I worked with, and it was a well-managed organization. With my focus on the petroleum industry, having Standard Oil listed on my resume was a prestigious plus, especially as I was a newcomer to California.

Additionally, having a set of objectives and having those personal goals recognized on my annual review was very rewarding to me. They were as follows:

- To provide excellent customer relations in addressing the needs of our credit card holders.

- To maintain my assigned accounts receivable at the best possible level.

- To excel in both letter writing and preparing departmental reports.

I was particularly pleased in meeting my third goal, knowing full well that the office manager was so persnickety about the quality of letters and reports. Prior to my review, a managerial assistant informed me that the office manager told the management team that I prepared the best quality documentation and letters in the office. To me, that compliment epitomized the equivalency of being insulted by the great Irish playwright, George Bernard Shaw.

I strongly believe that it was the office manager's favorable comments regarding my performance, along with those of the Southern belle, which caused the credit manager to occasionally stop by my unit. He would briefly chat with me; sometimes he would call me into his office for an exchange of ideas.

He would ask for my opinion on overall or general procedures and express his concerns about how to develop more effective follow-up tools within our data processing system. This struck me as being somewhat odd, as he never ventured too far from the administrative offices and his immediate managerial staff. The credit manager was definitely old school. He seemed to me to be a man who had worked his way up in the organization. Apparently, he had established an excellent reputation among his peers in the petroleum industry. On two or three occasions he sought my advice and thoughts regarding some specific concerns, which I viewed as being complimentary. During our discussions, he appeared very eager to hear my impressions on the topics that we covered.

On one occasion, I informed him that I planned on leaving Standard Oil very soon as I felt there was a long line before me. I was surprised that he displayed such pensiveness in discussing my leaving Standard Oil. As I definitely planned to leave their organization, he said he understood my feelings. He said, "Gus, Richfield Oil has recently lost several of their employees. I know Harry Swisher, their credit manager, and I would be most happy to assist you in seeking a position at Richfield Oil."

"Thank you; I shall keep Richfield in mind in seeking another position." Because of my initial meeting with Mr. Swisher, which I did not reveal to him, I remained noncommittal.

I had long decided that I would remain at Standard Oil just long enough to establish and strengthen my work experience as a newcomer to Los Angeles. As the work came so easily to me, I was able to devote my time to really refining my writing skills, strengthening my public relations skills, and developing and broadening my accounts receivable follow-up procedures.

I had time to interact with my colleagues and really help them develop their skills, placing me in somewhat of a teaching mode.

One young man who sat near me, upon returning from receiving his first review, said, "Gus, I got a great review and I informed the assistant credit manager that it was solely due to your tutelage."

"Wow, that is an unexpected compliment. What was his response?"

"Very favorable."

I left Standard Oil with no regrets, and I was anxious to continue working in the petroleum industry elsewhere. I quit cold turkey to seek other opportunities. It seemed incongruous that these college graduates—my co-workers—were learning much of their business acumen from a grade-school dropout. Some would individually ask to lunch with me privately so that they could address specific work issues and resolutions. One young man from the South said at lunch among the group, "Gus, you make more sense than anyone else in the department in discussing and addressing ongoing situations and issues. I go out of my way just to get your input."

Kind words; however, my scholastic achievements could still be listed on a blank piece of paper. I rationalized quitting my job cold turkey and fearlessly by stating, "If this is the only position available to me I should be unemployed and throwing in the towel." Up to this point in my life I had never been without work. I had voluntarily left each of my positions with flying colors and with expressions of gratitude and high marks for my performance from my employers. My irksome irritant was that "blank piece of paper" which may have been my greatest impetus to achieving vocational success. Perhaps this mental handicap was, in fact, a blessing in disguise? Unemployed but undaunted, I was ready for my next adventure.

10

Out of curiosity or vindictiveness—or both—I decided to bang on Harry Swisher's door once more. When I arrived in his office this time, he was extremely engaging and affable as he discussed his plight. Several of his credit men had moved on to another fast-moving credit card organization that was sweeping the country. He described his department and the general organization of the corporation and stated he was interested in having me go to work for him.

I said, "Mr. Swisher, I suggest that you contact the credit manager at Standard Oil for a reference."

"We have already spoken and you come to us with an excellence performance history and nothing more need be said."

"Thank you."

"Mr. Munro, I am really happy to have you join our organization."

While I never pursued the issue, I am certain Mr. Swisher had no recollection of our first meeting. After the negativity of our first encounter, I changed my mind about him very quickly. I was so pleased that I had come back for the second time.

I was immediately assigned to the credit card unit and informed that I would be responsible for their heaviest-volume unit. It seemed that this had been decided because of my prior experience, and perhaps they were running me through a test.

After I had been there for about four months, Mr. Swisher stopped by my unit and informed me in the presence of my assistant that there would be a staff meeting in thirty minutes. He requested that, at this meeting, I impart to the troops the rules of the game. He stated, "You have an excellent background and I want you to instruct the credit men in productive ways to use the telephone, and to write letters effectively. I want you to provide any other tools and information that will help make them more effective in the collection of their accounts receivable."

"Mr. Swisher, I shall do my best."

"Because of your experience, you have a greater workload than the others and your figures are very impressive for just being here a short time."

"Is there a time limit for my presentation?"

"No, keep it open."

"I like doing questions and answers as I go along, is that okay?"

"Perfect!"

Normally, in making such a presentation, I would have preferred a couple of days' notice so I could prepare. I also would have preferred to use a flipchart to keep the discussion on target.

After Mr. Swisher left my office, my assistant, a considerate lady, said, "He isn't giving you much notice to make such a broad presentation."

"That isn't the problem. The problem is a new kid on the block telling everyone else the game plan."

The meeting went very well. I received tremendous support and participation on the salient points that I had addressed—by the senior staff and managers. And I perceived that Mr. Swisher was delighted with my presentation.

To a newcomer with industry background, they were very supportive as I addressed their concerns. After the meeting, those men in the units who were my peers stopped by individually to see me, wondering why I had been selected to address the meeting. They all knew I demonstrated low-key, in-office fraternization from top to bottom. I was not too surprised that they stopped by inquisitively.

Paradoxically, through no fault of my own, after our very rocky start, I turned out to be Harry Swisher's fair-haired boy. And he turned out to be a very dear man, and so kind to me. It was certainly an unexpected turn of events. It was a joyful experience for me. In reviewing the end result, I realized that all of the negativity I had harbored after our first encounter had eventually been a total waste of time.

One of Mr. Swisher's closest associates pulled me aside one day and said, "Gus, Mr. Swisher thinks you are wonderful and he speaks of you in glowing terms. He is really pleased with you and believes you will have a very successful and rewarding career at Richfield Oil Corporation."

"You mean I'm like the teacher's pet?"

"You got it, Gus!"

After a few months, I received a promotion to the credit card approval unit and I stayed there for a short period of time. In less than two years, I was promoted to the wholesale unit that addressed the needs of all of our Richfield Oil branch distribution centers. An agent and staff operated each office and they provided products for our service stations, small and large business accounts, farm and agriculturally related accounts, and major commercial and industrial enterprises.

Geographically, our office was responsible only for Southern California, which was divided into three parts. I was assigned, along with two other young men, to this unit and we each had a private secretarial assistant. A certain amount of travel was involved in visiting our agencies, who were key to our organization and many of their major accounts. My area covered parts of Los Angeles and areas located up the coast to San Luis Obispo. It was a very desirable and scenic territory and, in those days, somewhat sparsely populated. It was a wonderful place and time.

This position was equivalent to the last position I had held at British American Oil Company. Since my arrival to Los Angeles it had taken me almost five years to get back to a comparable position. It was a much more demanding position than the one at British American Oil. California was growing by leaps and bounds. New construction companies and related industries were sprouting up everywhere. Keeping a competitive edge, we were assessing many of their new accounts with somewhat very limited historical documentation.

In some cases we were approving the accounts based on the key individuals involved and their current and projected work-in-progress worksheets. We obtained key evaluation reports and summaries from our agents and sales personnel. Comprehensive assessments were determined and the final decisions were sagaciously made. I had tremendous admiration for the key personnel in both marketing and finance in this organization. I thoroughly enjoyed being operationally involved to a lesser degree in the informational gathering process.

Mr. Swisher retired around the time I was promoted to the wholesale unit and I reported to (another) Jack, one of Mr. Swisher's assistant credit managers. Jack was eight years older than I. He was extremely bright and had an inquiring mind for detail. He was small in stature but very wiry. His avocation was volunteering his services to the Sierra Madre Rescue Service. He would jump out of helicopters and do mountain terrain rescues on the weekends and sometime weekday evenings.

He was a total contradiction—extremely loyal and meticulous in his performance, and a total rebel in terms of working with the bigwigs at the home office. He was a handful, but no one questioned his ability. He had a slide rule (excuse the pun) never more than a foot away from him, which he used incessantly.

He and I would make business stops and he would always drive in his Volkswagen like a madman, cutting into lanes between huge trucks and I would be screaming from the top of my voice in fear. Each time we got back to the office I would say, "Never again!" Upon our return he would relate the experiences of our joy rides to the group and they would scream with laughter at my expense. He called me by my initials, AR (my full name is Angus Roy Munro). The troops loved to hear his AR stories and AR was happy to have survived those joy rides! During one of our outings, Jack and I were heading up north to Santa Barbara. He informed me that he and his sister were the legatees on a vast number of acres in the Agoura area, the far outskirts of the San Fernando Valley. It was impressively beautiful rural acreage and Jack believed that he and his sister would be well endowed in their senior years. The San Fernando Valley and lands to the west were starting to expand in housing developments and he felt assured they were sitting on a real estate gold mine. It was a legacy worth several million dollars.

During this period, I was also attending UCLA and I had taken a course in real estate law. When I started working with Jack, our department was very involved in real estate activities pertaining to our agents and service station lessees. In practicality, Jack was definitely much better than the course. He took me to a title company and went through the process of title searching and everything relating to real estate practices including conditional sales agreements, and the like. He took me into the field and covered the practical applications in terms of what forms to use and the various steps that needed to be taken to achieve the end result. He was casually bright, a great mentor, and so composed in his educational instructions to me.

I had been in the wholesale unit less than three months when he and the new credit manager asked that I bring all of my trays of accounts to the manager's office. Wholesale accounts still remained on a manually operated billing machine system. They informed me discreetly that the person next to me, who had been there for some time, was not able to provide the appropriate documentation or status on the accounts under his stewardship. I reviewed my accounts, agency by agency, and, when I was half way through, they looked at each other and said, "You're fine."

I had long since learned the importance of ongoing follow-up procedures that assured no surprises. I never wanted to find myself in an untenable position.

After I had been in the unit for several months, one morning Jack asked we three senior representatives to come to his office as he wanted to discuss a very serious problem. He addressed the complex situation that required both data and ongoing follow-up, and I quickly answered with a full solution and all agreed.

About ten minutes later he called me into his office and told me to close the door. He looked at me very seriously and poignantly said, "Never tell me what you think of my work or my general performance by making a comparison between you and me."

I told him, "Your work is great and your performance is exceptional. What are we discussing here?"

"I had been pondering over this problem we just discussed for days and was unable to arrive at a solution. You answered it immediately with a perfect conclusion."

"We all throw out ideas that others help to resolve. It's a two-way street."

"Gus, why are you so critical of yourself? I could not compete with your high work standards. No one in this department is in your league, including me. You are a perfectionist."

"Oh, is that the reason you take me on those frightening joy rides, to scare the shit out of this self-critical perfectionist?"

"AR, who can win with you?"

It was a touching moment, but deep down my self-esteem was still cemented in the realization that I had dropped out of school and had served unappreciatively, relegated to clean up after my father's parties and poker games. Old scars heal slowly—or resurface and fester.

On a few occasions, I spent a little time in our corporate office—the magnificent gold domed building. I met with our general corporate credit manager, who was a very friendly individual. He was concerned with maintaining good customer relations and expanding our marketing activities in Southern California in both wholesale and retail services. I mentioned to him that I was concerned when layoffs occurred at Lockheed and other aircraft and defense plants that would affect our credit card customers. I discussed our policies and procedures from our standpoint and from the standpoint of a customer who had suddenly become unemployed for the first time and had a family to support and bills to pay. This issue was a key concern to me in terms of retaining our customers' goodwill when settlement issues were involved.

I gave the general corporate credit manager some of my thoughts about addressing these types of situations—thoughts that would be beneficial to the company and to the customer. I had also done some random research within the organization that seemed to impress him. In my meetings with him, we never planned an agenda, we just carried on off-the-cuff conversations. I sort of got the feeling he was attempting to get to know me better and enjoyed our unfettered exchange of ideas.

Socially, rumors were that the general corporate credit manager was quite a character. Apparently, he was president of an executive managers' association, and both he and his wife attended the organization's annual formal function, which took place at a large hotel. When he and his wife arrived at the function, they were presented and then they began to walk down the grand staircase to greet the awaiting members and their spouses. The story went that they were both more than slightly inebriated. About halfway down the stairs, his wife fell and he didn't even notice—he was blindly looking straight ahead preparing to receive the other guests. They said it was an absolute riot, and, fortunately, the wife was not hurt, just somewhat embarrassed. I can only say that it must have been a sobering experience for both, and a sight to behold.

The general corporate credit manager offered a member of his church a position in our office. She was the daughter-in-law of the former California Governor Olson. While Olson was in office his wife had died and his daughter-in-law had assumed her late mother-in-law's role as first lady. After the governor left office, the daughter-in-law and her husband divorced. Because of that, her first job after being first lady was working in a restaurant as a hostess/cashier. She told us that the first Friday at work a truck driver came up to her and said, "Hey, babe, how about a date tonight?" Apparently he didn't recognize her as the former first lady, but she was still a good scout and graciously declined his offer. She had a pragmatic sense of being and went with the flow.

She worked arduously and had a great sense of humor. She had remained best friends with actress Loretta Young. Not uncommonly, her other celebrity and socialite friends apparently abandoned her after her divorce, when her social status dropped. She was blessed with a very realistic and down-to-earth approach to life. She told us that when she and her husband were first married they went dancing at the Coconut Grove along with former starlet Joan Crawford. Her husband said to her, "Stay away from Crawford; she is too wild!" One day she said to me with great humor, "Today I am a clerk at Richfield Oil and Joan Crawford is on the board of directors at Pepsi Cola and a renowned world-famous actress!"

The general corporate credit manager hired an attorney who also worked in the regional office. He could best be described as the personification of a Damon Runyon character. He was diminutive in stature, extremely frail, and, unfortunately, visibly very crippled in his upper torso and back. Sadly, this had been due to an accident during his infancy. His babysitter had taken him for a stroll and decided to take a shortcut back home. While attempting to climb over a neighbor's fence, she dropped him. She then failed to notify his parents in a timely fashion of this incident, thus, causing a lifetime of physical disabilities for this man.

However, aside from his physical impairment, he was quite brilliant and occupationally extremely successful. He did not outwardly dwell on his misfortunate and obvious handicaps. His avocation was solely the Hollywood Racetrack. He loved to gamble and loved the horses. I would often see him at the bus stop on Wilshire Boulevard and I would stop and drive him to work. I would occasionally drop him off after work, too. And most of his conversation related to his positive and negative moments at the racetrack.

His duty at Richfield was to perform the final review of all applications for credit cards and/or commercial businesses that had been denied by our credit department. He believed every denied application could represent missed dollars and he was very diligent, yet pragmatic, in reviewing each denial to see if it could be approved. If he approved the application, he indicated his approval with a shaky *S*.

I always viewed the *S* as a marginal approval, and, when I worked accounts for potential problem situations, I would review the initial customer file to see if the approval contained the shaky *S*.

While working in the approval unit, I referred an application to another colleague for his evaluation, as I felt ambivalent in terms of approving/rejecting the application. He looked at it and simply made a shaky *S* and passed it back to me.

I thought to myself, *There are some things that I would rather not know about nefariously watering down the system.*

Our management decided to celebrate a special occasion. It wasn't designated as an awards event, but rather a "Rewards Theme"—an appreciation event. All employees, along with their spouses, were invited to attend. The dinner was held at the Smokehouse restaurant in Burbank, across the street from Warner Brothers Studio. My wife Rose and I both frequented and loved the restaurant and we were looking forward to attending the event.

After dinner, there were a couple of appreciative presentational comments and after-dinner speeches and comments by our leadership. They wanted the evening to be informal and fun and they were personalizing comments to my colleagues—this one is crazy about baseball, the other loves football, and so on. About some people, they mentioned one-liners, or humorous events, but nothing relating to their work or performance—they kept it light. I was waiting my turn and expected comments about my being a tennis or beach bum. One speaker began, "And then there is Gus Munro. What could we say about him that we haven't already heard? All joking aside, I believe one word says it all: outstanding!"

Frankly, I was slightly embarrassed and I kept my demeanor low-key for the rest of the evening. Driving home with my wife we had the following exchange:

She began, "When they were making those frivolous comments about your colleagues, I wondered what they had in mind for you?"

"Me too!"

"Gus, you work for a large corporation and they think very highly of you to make such comments."

"It was nice."

"That's not my point. You have been very successful—at the CPR, British American Oil, Standard Oil, and now Richfield. I am certain that they are currently grooming you for an even higher position down the road. It is time to wake up!"

"What is your point?"

"Today and for several years, you have not been a fourteen-year-old, grade-school dropout. You are a successful, up-and-coming executive. Get over it and get with it!"

"Rose, I have heard of a similar case. There's a successful top executive in the banking business who is another grade-school dropout—sort of another Gus Munro with the same associated feelings. Perhaps you should find him and tell him to get over it and get with it. Apparently, his wife had not been as encouraging toward him."

"There you go again, hiding behind humor." This is an example of why I loved my wife so much then and continue to do so today. However, sadly, I found no harmonic balance between my love for her and my impatience for some of her dislikable tendencies. There were two powerful emotions going in both directions—simultaneously. I simply could not singularly resolve this ongoing dilemma in our relationship.

Despite receiving laudatory comments, I still inwardly believed that I was a fraudulent grade-school dropout and someday the posse would catch up with me and expose me for what I was. I did not however, steal that student's fountain pen. I tried but couldn't rationalize that, due to circumstantial misfortune, I had taken a divergent path, working diligently to improve myself in every possible way to arrive at the same destination with the others that had chosen traditional education. I totally dismissed my wife's praiseworthy comments, because I knew she truly loved me. I could not dismiss the thought that she was a very bright and an accomplished, up-front person. I was a supervisor, while she was a branch manager at the CPR and she had given me good guidance.

I was mindful in attending meetings and special sessions in which guest speakers were introduced by clearly stating their backgrounds both educationally and professionally. Managers usually consider educational background when considering employees for promotion.

I did have a concern about being promoted to the corporate office—not for the initial position, but for what might happen thereafter. Being a grade-school dropout was not a plus. One could argue that I had been extremely successful; however, others could say I had probably reached my level of competence—or incompetence, as in the Peter Principle ("In a hierarchy, every employee tends to rise the level of his incompetence." Laurance J. Peter, *The Peter Principle*, 1968.) We all live semi-sealed in our own little emotional boxes.

If person A holds a senior position, he is closing the door for person B, who has a stronger background and who should assume the role of person A to ensure a natural continuum up the ladder. If person B is promoted, the choice for person A would be to return to the lower trenches or leave the organization. My problem in the entire scheme of promotional considerations within the organization included these thoughts. No one person, with the exception of my manager at the T. Eaton Company, knew of my limited educational background. He was a grade-school dropout, too—a very polished one, I may add.

I held very demanding positions that required my full attention, and I was only able to allocate a very small portion of my time for selective courses at the university. I strongly focused on accepting any challenging assignments with alacrity to further my interest and to provide me with more additional empirical education. With all of my success and recognition, I still felt I was in limbo land waiting for the hammer to drop. In totality, I felt branded—a dropout with an *F* for failure.

It was informally brought to my attention that, as soon as an older member of the department in the corporate office retired, I would be scheduled for his position at the home office. The position I had at Richfield Oil was both demanding and very rewarding; however, I did not see myself transferring to the home office and reporting directly to the general corporate credit manager. The position was prestigious and I was flattered, but I also was concerned. However, I was also keenly aware that turning down an opportunity for advancement does not set well in the corporate structure: pass and thou shalt be passed over.

My decision could have limited my career in terms of other opportunities within the organization. All of these thoughts came at me at the same time. Up to this point, they had been back-burner issues and often suppressed due to my heavy work schedule and immediate responsibilities. Now they were all on the front burner. In looking at the entire picture—the pros and cons—I thought maybe it was time I considered a new career in a new field.

I learned that there was speculation that the Atlantic Refining Corporation and Richfield Oil Corporation were planning a merger. I realized that, if the merger materialized, things would change. I was strongly considering leaving the petroleum business. I had a meeting with Jack to share my superficial thoughts. He stated that I had been in this business for nine years and, if I left, I would simply just go elsewhere but remain in the same industry, which made no sense to him. He was visibly concerned at the prospects of my changing employment. Because of that, during this transitional thought process, I decided to keep any comments on the subject to myself. Needless to say, he was not privy to the many concerns and considerations running through my mind. At this late date, I certainly wasn't going to tell him that he was strongly promoting a grade-school dropout who was loaded with anxiety in terms of future promotions.

At Richfield, I worked closely with the marketing department and the director of marketing. I would send to marketing copies of financial credit and history reports that I would obtain from Dun and Bradstreet and other agencies for updating purposes or for new business. This was a very routine situation.

On one occasion, I researched a possible new account for marketing and I sent the reports and a memorandum stating my opinion on the advantages of working with this new organization.

I viewed my input as a positive gesture and not an intrusive one.

I immediately received a terse response from the director of marketing stating that he made the marketing decisions and my position was obtaining the financial reports.

This was a negative repercussion—a new experience for me. Strangely, after that incident, he began to rely on my assistance and became less condescending in our exchange of information. He would go out of his way to be cordial and actually brief me on certain accounts that he would approve or with which he had some concern, which was very complimentary.

He assertively became very up front with me, and communicated in a straightforward manner with no BS, which I most admired. The outcome was that he became extremely friendly and very relaxed with me. I perceived that he liked our exchanges and respected my viewpoints. In retrospect, I realized that I had actually brought myself to his attention by sending him that memorandum regarding the merits of a prospective customer.

When he learned that I was thinking of leaving the organization, he offered me a position in marketing. He made it very clear that this was a very complimentary gesture on his part and admitted he was very impressed with my performance. They virtually never obtained sales recruits from within the company. I did decline his offer, but it was great to know that we had developed a good rapport.

I did believe I had strong marketing proclivities, but I lacked the gift of gab in working with clients. Those positions called for taking the clients to lunch and other forms of fraternization that absolutely had no appeal to me.

I finally decided that I definitely wanted to make a career change. One of my Richfield colleagues had previously accepted a clerical position in a large hospital in West Los Angeles while he worked on his master's degree. Occasionally, we commuted together as we both lived in Santa Monica. During those trips, he frequently and emphatically mentioned that I should consider a career in healthcare; namely, in hospital administration. He thought my personality and professional background would really blend well in that field. He was scholastically quite brilliant and I respected his observations and assessments. I frankly had no interest in healthcare or continuing credit management and I was totally perplexed about what course of action to take. I had always worked so diligently and had been so focused on my work responsibilities that I could never see beyond my desk. Based on that and my impulsive nature, I decided to leave Richfield and be free to pursue other opportunities.

Strangely enough, with my limited educational background and deep-seated insecurities, I truthfully never ever really worried about being out of work. Jack was extremely unhappy with my decision to leave, as were the other management staff and my colleagues. They thought I was bonkers for leaving a position with an almost assured bright future there or at the home office. They freely condemned the idea of my leaving cold turkey.

In the process, I did elevate my decision by knowing that I had been very successful there. I strongly believed that I had made a fulfilling contribution within my department and the organization. And I knew that I was well liked and respected by all, including the director of marketing.

When my successor was selected, he and Jack stopped by to chat with me. I informed my replacement, "I would like to take you on a tour of the organization and introduce you to key persons who will be able to help you when certain situations arise."

And Jack chimed in by facetiously saying, "I'd like to join you—maybe I'll pick-up some pointers." We toured the regional office from top to bottom. In introducing my replacement, I would state what that person's role was, and how and when interaction was essential. I would cite specific examples.

I frankly believe that Jack was as much impressed with the tour as my replacement. He jokingly interjected comments, such as, "I didn't know that!" while simultaneously carrying a shameful grin.

I explained the importance of knowing what others do in the various departments, as one never knows how helpful one can be to the other. When the tour was over, Jack made several laudatory remarks about me to my successor in my presence. I believe Jack was unequivocally my greatest fan ever, and expressed his appreciation for my general work performance. He himself was no slouch.

One of my favorite colleagues, who left Richfield at about the same time I did, became a CPA and joined his father's practice. We continued to socialize thereafter. He would mention performing audits in various organizations, and, if they were faced with some difficult internal problems, he would say to himself, "Gus Munro, where are you? You are badly needed in this organization." He would state it more humorously than I. Being recognized by your colleagues may possibly be more rewarding than kudos from your superiors; however, I inwardly thought such laudatory praise was wasted on this secretive enigmatic dropout.

The day prior to my departure date, my colleagues arranged a farewell party for me at a popular Irish pub and grill near the office. I viewed this gathering just as an informal small get-together and didn't ask my wife to accompany me. However, our group took over most of the place, as virtually everyone showed up. Their kind gesture of participation really pleased me. One lady, who had assisted me within the department, apparently had an ongoing somewhat mad crush on me, which I had ignored. It became obvious to other members of the department and I received frequent not-so-subtle teasing reminders from my colleagues.

At the gathering, she sat close to me at a long table accompanied by her fiancé. They were both slightly older than I, but an attractive couple, and, fortunately, he was unaware of her supposed interest in me, which could have just been superficial.

He was extremely engaging and a somewhat dominating conversationalist and focused his thoughts directly toward me throughout the entire evening. He stated his lady had spoken so highly of my performance at work. He said that he was in business and he would hire me immediately if I would accept a position he could offer me. While this was only a spur-of-the-moment situation, my interest was still piqued in anticipation of his proposal.

He said very compellingly, "I own two very lucrative gay bars in the area and I would love you to run one of them for me!"

I said, "But, I'm not gay and I'm not a bartender!"

He responded, "With your good looks, who cares? We could make so much money just having you on the premises!"

After the initial shock, my sense of humor took over and I thought it was quite funny.

My colleagues at the table, overhearing his proposal, roared knowing my personal moral values relating to the bar scene and my dedicated business background. He spent the whole evening trying to get me to consider his proposal. Frankly, it may have been a better proposal than learning that his lady had a crush on me. I wondered if she may have been the instigator of his plan.

On my last day at Richfield, to accommodate my successor, who also took his work seriously, I completed a total review of all of my open accounts and left applicable helpful salient notes. I had gotten so engrossed in this project that, before leaving, I had joined our janitorial staff for coffee at their midnight break. "Hi guys!" I'd said, "Today is my last day at Richfield. After I have coffee with you I am going to clear my desk and leave. This has been a long day for me, but I had to get everything in order before leaving."

"Oh no! We'll miss you," said one.

Another guy questioned, "Where do you go from here?"

"I am not certain. I want to take a couple of weeks off and then start looking around—maybe try working in another field."

"You'll be fine—you work hard and everyone likes you and we'll miss you."

"Take your time and find a good job and be happy."

I inquired, "What happened to your co-worker—the young man who cleaned our offices?"

"Who was that?"

"You know him—they called him 'Mother' or something?"

All hell broke loose as they went berserk, roaring with laughter at this uninformed transplanted Canadian. Frankly, I didn't know what was happening.

They looked at me, pointing, as if saying, "This guy is nuts or naive or both."

Finally, one man replied, "We knew him. His first name was 'Mother'; his surname was 'F——r.'"

Laughingly, I said, "No wonder the poor guy moved on—you are bad. He worked so hard." We all, while still laughing hard, got up shook hands and said farewell. What a sendoff—and they were a jolly crew of guys. I was so dumb, I had never heard of that expression before. It was so funny, and I left the building on my day of departure laughing like hell. I laughed all the way home to Santa Monica over that coffee break with those guys. It was a great ending and a humorous reward.

A few weeks later, I was driving along Wilshire Boulevard en route to my new position. Suddenly I realized that the man who succeeded me at Richfield was driving alongside me. At each stoplight he would laugh and yell words of gratitude for leaving such great documentation for him. Additionally, he commented on how well I had maintained the files. Appreciative people make everything all worthwhile, and I felt so good that day hearing his words.

11

After leaving Richfield Oil, I decided to leave the healthcare option open. I read an advertisement in the *Los Angeles Times* for an open position for an accounts receivable manager at a large and prestigious hospital in Los Angeles. I applied for the opening and, after completing two extensive interviews, I was offered the position. However, I was slightly hesitant and cautiously deferred my decision temporarily. I had some concerns and decided to see what other opportunities were available before saying "yea" or "nay." They were interested enough to accept my temporary postponement of commitment.

In the process, I stopped at another prominent hospital and spoke with one of their administrative executives. It was an informal meeting, but, when he learned of my background, he encouraged me to seek a position in healthcare. He spoke very enthusiastically about the advantages of having a career in hospital administration. He thought my qualifications could be transferred without difficulty to the healthcare industry. He said it was a very innovative period for hospitals, and my business acumen would be beneficial in the healthcare setting. There were no open positions at that hospital, but I accepted ebulliently his encouraging words regarding hospital administration and my background.

I had also been informed that a leading record company in Hollywood had an interesting intermediate open position. I arranged an interview with one of their key persons. I wanted to leave my options open so I could calmly explore all possibilities—and avoid any spur-of-the-moment decisions.

My interview at the record company was with the person whom the applicant would report to in the organization—a nice woman, mid-fifties, plain appearance and dress, but "hip," pleasantly spoken, and she greeted me warmly.

"So, Mr. Munro, I see from your application that you have been in the petroleum industry for several years. What brings you to our organization?"

"I believe I need a new focus and a revitalized direction in my career path. I have been very successful and I want to consider other options—perhaps something new. Your open position sounds very interesting and challenging to me."

"I assume from your background that you have had a lot of responsibilities, and that is usually associated with a heavy workload to process."

"Very true. I am sort of like an octopus. I naturally enjoy being involved with many projects—as well as assisting others in the process—all to accomplish a common goal. Working closely with our district agents and our internal and external sales force on marketing and other issues to increase their volumes is but one example."

"The record industry is hectic and there is a tremendous need for drive to keep on top of this competitive business. Our staff must produce and excel."

"Hard work is my second nature and I welcome innovating projects and new challenges. I initially try to discern the bread-and-butter, basic issues and how to expand from that foundation. If that makes sense?"

"You present yourself very favorably. You are well groomed, very good looking, and articulate."

"Thank you!"

"I believe you are the kind of person I would love to have on my team and really groom you for bigger and better opportunities within the organization."

"That sounds great!"

"Mr. Munro, although I am being complimentary, unfortunately, there isn't a chance in hell that I would hire you!"

Really taken back, I replied, "Why, may I ask?"

"There is no question in terms of your qualifications based on your background; however, you wouldn't be happy here. From the top to the bottom of this organization, it's the F-word this and F-word that. My assessment is that you are an excellent candidate, but would have an aversion for this somewhat uncouth setting—which is complimentary to you."

I appealingly stated, "Well, should we consider the old adage, 'When in Rome?'"

Laughingly, she said, "No, I don't think so!"

"Believe me, if everything else fits, I could do it." (I was silently thinking that this exchange of dialogue seemed so unprecedented.)

"Frankly, Mr. Munro, I like your good manners and the fine qualities you exhibit. Go where you will be most appreciated with those good attributes. It's not here."

"Thanks, I enjoyed meeting you and I must accept your decision."

"You will have no problem finding the right position. Good luck!"

I must confess, in later pondering and revisiting this scenario, I was quite surprised and actually shocked. I enjoyed my meeting with her. I thought she, personally, would have been great to work with as a straightforward lady. I wasn't really disappointed; I had just had a very interesting and somewhat intriguing interview with a lady with obvious integrity and, apparently, great foresight and perceptiveness.

I had had a minor overnight surgical procedure at The Hospital of the Good Samaritan while I was still employed at Standard Oil, so I decided to apply for a position at that hospital. Instead of stopping by their personnel department to ascertain possible open positions or to complete an application, I simply called the personnel department. I spoke with the assistant to the personnel manager, who seemed interested in my telephone conversation with her and she, sight unseen, arranged the interview. When we met, she informed me that I had projected myself very favorably over the telephone and I sounded like a good candidate for their hospital. At the time of my interview, I had not declined the other hospital's offer, though it was decisively a front-burner issue. During my second interview at The Hospital of the Good Samaritan, I informed the chief financial officer (CFO) that the other position was still pending, awaiting my decision.

The CFO informed me that she was interested in creating a new position for me; however, they had some loose ends to address in getting me onboard.

I started working at The Hospital of the Good Samaritan on June 1, 1964, two years prior to the implementation of the Medicare and Medicaid programs. I did not realize at the time that it was a very transitional and controversial period in the healthcare field. The major insurance companies were attempting to address the needs of the senior population through private plans. They were hoping to eliminate and/or prolong the feasibility of governmental intervention into the healthcare industry.

The Hospital of the Good Samaritan at that time was considered one of the top five hospitals in the United States. That classification was based on their outstanding and prestigious medical staff. Every physician on staff was a specialist. There were no general practitioners practicing medical care there. That was quite outstanding for the early 1960s. The hospital was renowned for providing medical care to numerous movie stars and other prominent persons. It had been an established haven for celebrities, constantly, over the years.

I was hired with the title of consultant; I was based in business services. I had total responsibility for our accounts receivable with involvement in all non-medical departments. I was actually given a broad range in terms of my duties. I was just freely playing it by ear and fitting the pieces together as I moved along. This open structure was befitting to my open-boundaries approach—go where needed. It became abundantly clear to me that this would definitely be a hands-on operation in terms of my role.

I immediately got involved with patients and/or their family members in terms of financial assessments, insurance issues, and so on. To learn the operation, I immersed myself in all phases of insurance and other third-party payer issues, which included confirmation of benefits and the expediting of payment for our services. In those days, the leaders in healthcare were Blue Cross and Blue Shield of California. Both Blue Cross and Blue Shield sent their representatives to hospitals routinely to address any billing or policy issues. Blue Shield mainly focused on the physician fees; however, they, too, offered hospital plans. Both organizations accepted leadership in the training of hospital personnel, as they were responsible for the majority of contracts at that time.

Many other insurance companies had large contracts as well; however, the majority of hospital admissions were through Blue Cross. Adherence to their training manuals was essential in obtaining timely payments. In the early 1960s, prior to the advent of the government plans of Medicare and Medicaid, insurance plan verification and billing were less complicated than they are today. It was a natural transition when the Medicare and Medicaid programs were enacted in July 1966 that Blue Cross would be in the vanguard of those administrating those programs, along with Aetna and a few other larger insurance corporations.

I soon learned that it was imperative to develop and maintain good working relationships with our physicians and their office personnel. I found myself meeting and working with many persons from all walks of life relating to hospital costs and insurance issues for them individually and/or for their family members. Regardless of a person's individual station in life, when addressing hospital issues, there is a defined commonality in terms of both concern and outcome. It was an extremely rewarding situation for me and also often required the involvement of the physicians and/or their office staff. Working closely like this, many physicians over the years have requested I call them by their Christian or first name; I have declined, and have afforded them the title that they worked so tenaciously to obtain.

Fortunately, the hospital was expanding their pre-admission unit that was a part of the admitting office. They had just hired a coordinator, Rosemary, to run the unit. She had been in hospital administration all of her working years. She had been an assistant to the administrator at a smaller hospital. She was close to receiving a master's degree in healthcare and she taught me the ropes from top to bottom. She was a few years older than I, very intelligent, and extremely hardworking. She also had a tremendous sense of humor. Both enthusiastic, we instantly became great friends. When an anomaly occurred she would pitch in and help me. We had lunch together every day and we developed an ongoing rapport as she taught me the business. It was a very prestigious organization and we were both informed on numerous occasions that we represented the hospital favorably.

Responding to a knock on my office door, I might expect key executives of brokerage houses, heads of department stores, top banking personnel, movie representatives, and celebrities (and many from a bygone era).

They were all incredibly respectful to me and freely discussed their concerns. Also, they were extremely appreciative of my assistance and intervention in resolving insurance or other related issues. A very prominent brokerage president, when leaving my office, said that his private secretary instructed him to personally see me regarding his wife's hospitalization. She had told him, "Mr. Munro will take care of everything, so just see him."

He smiled and said, "My secretary is never wrong and it has been a pleasure meeting you."

That evening at home I informed my wife, "I met your president today."

One prominent retail president had a college-age daughter who had a preexisting condition. It needed to be monitored and kept under control. Due to her condition, she loved being hospitalized. The daughter resided with his estranged wife and I kept in close touch with the father, as he was responsible for her financial care above insurance. He was grateful for my intervention to limit the patient's hospital stays in working with the physician and hospital medical personnel. The patient loved the attention and tried to prolong her confinement by attempting to hoodwink our staff. The father sought my assistance in having his daughter discharged in a timely manner and he freely expressed his gratitude on several occasions for my ongoing participation. This is but one example of personal intervention in working with families and our medical staff.

The top administration of the hospital, at that time, had long been staffed by women only, a situation that was uncommon in the '60s. It was a prestigious organization, but somewhat infused with elitism. Plainly put, the staff was prone to snobbishness. The CFO announced to my department prior to my arrival, that I was to be called "Mr. Munro" and never to be addressed by my Christian name. During my private orientation with the CFO, she instructed me never to leave my office without wearing my jacket. Being a shirtsleeve type, I found that ruling difficult; however, I accepted it based on my respect and admiration for her. Rosemary and I were snobbishly instructed, as management personnel, not to fraternize with non-management employees on lunch or coffee breaks. Both being down to earth and outgoing, we found that edict hard to swallow—commiseration being our safety net. My wife and I would attend parties with other employees and she would say, "Don't call him 'Mr. Munro' away from work. He's just plain 'Gus.'"

The staff members would respond, "If we start calling him 'Gus' we could forget at work and really get into trouble for not calling him 'Mr. Munro.'"

As I mentioned, the original Brown Derby Restaurant—the famous one shaped like the hat—was across the street from my former office at Richfield Oil, and I had enjoyed taking district agents and clients there for lunch. The owner of that famous restaurant had another restaurant in Hollywood that was also patronized by the movie colony. Myself, I preferred "the hat." The owner, who had created the famous Cobb Salad—appropriately named after him, became very ill while I was at Good Samaritan, and his wife stopped by to see me several times.

She was attractive and statuesque and was always accompanied by two rather burly, but very well dressed, gentlemen. I wasn't certain of their roles—were they combined business associates and bodyguards? The three were always very pleasant; she was very commanding and businesslike. She had apparently been best friend to actress Carole Lombard, who tragically died in an air crash while married to Clark Gable. Mrs. Cobb was interesting, appreciative, and gracious, but sadly her husband was seriously ill.

I met several celebrates at the hospital, and being an ardent old movie buff, I found these meetings interesting. I particularly liked Mrs. Cobb, but it is sad meeting nice folks under trying circumstances. However, they do appreciate being treated kindly and receiving meaningful services to lessen their burden. It was an important ongoing placatory role for me to fulfill.

The main or branch offices of many insurance companies, as well as our physicians' medical offices, were located within the nearby downtown area. I worked closely with the key personnel in these businesses. Periodically, I would invite them for lunch and would ask them where they would like to dine. Virtually, one hundred percent would say, "Let's go to your hospital coffee shop—their food is so good." One of my insurance colleagues always ordered the breakfast waffle for lunch. During those years I believe the hospital had six or seven qualified dieticians on staff to serve the dietary needs of our patients. The food was excellent, even in our cafeteria, and seniors residing in nearby converted hotels took their meals there daily as the food was reasonably priced and balanced and nutritious. Most of those seniors were also, befittingly, patients of our medical staff.

When I arrived at the hospital, only a short period of time had passed since they had converted from a manual to a computerized billing system. With major changes on the horizon regarding the proposed introduction to the federal and state implementation of the Medicare and Medicaid programs, further computerization was anticipated. Both our CFO and her assistant CFO were CPAs and their background experiences had been in manual billing procedures. As computerization was in its infancy, there was a tremendous growing need for experts in the new computer field and ongoing advancing technological era.

The hospital hired a candidate whose background covered the conversion of state programs in a northwestern state. Seemingly, this individual, who was in his late thirties, had developed a great resume that covered computer sciences, and the hospital was elated to be able to obtain his services. I must preface that he was hired as an employee and not a consultant.

While we were an individual medical facility, it was a tremendous expense to obtain a singular full-service system. Because of his expertise, hospital administration and the board of directors, without hesitancy, approved his recommendations pertaining to the proposed new upgraded installation. I surmised that the CFO, known for her commanding leadership, along with her competent assistant, felt intimidated in having to take a back seat in the decision making regarding the advanced computer installation.

Further, as this new computer specialist had recently come onboard, they didn't know him personally that well; however, he did have a verified background in this new rising field. Finally, all of the plant and equipment necessary for the new installation was approved and ordered. We had anticipated delivery date.

One day, upon returning to her office after an administrative luncheon meeting, the CFO called me and said, "Mr. Munro, please come to my office immediately." When I arrived, she said, "Sit down. I don't know where to start, I am so upset."

"What happened?"

"As you know, with the advent of these new government programs, we have had to upgrade and enhance our total billing and accounting system."

"Yes, I fully understand."

"We felt very fortunate in acquiring the services of our computer specialist, who came to us with a very impressive background and with verified credentials."

"I agree. This is a big project and undertaking for this medical center."

"Yes, and every recommendation proposed by the specialist was approved and set in place. Now we are awaiting delivery and installation. Mr. Munro, I returned to my office from lunch today and found a letter of resignation from the specialist sitting on my desk!"

"What? You can't be serious!"

She was furious, and continued, "To add insult to injury, he even telephoned me after I returned from my lunch meeting to ask if I had received his letter."

"I can't believe this! As bad as the situation appears, the very least he could have done would be to be man enough to meet with you privately and address the situation. I have no respect for him just dropping the ball and running off."

"Precisely!"

"What are your thoughts in terms of a replacement?"

"Mr. Munro, I want your input on Miss J, our other hired assistant, who has been working with him."

"Fortunately, they came from different directions and they have had no prior joint affiliations. Frankly, she has been working in depth with our people on preliminary issues and they all seem to like and respect her."

"I share your view. I want to get moving on a concrete alternative plan, as I have to pass all of this information 'upstairs' and then along to the board. This situation places me in an untenable position as I supported that man in fulfilling all of his requests."

"Needless to say, I share your concerns and confidentiality. I believe Miss J is our candidate."

A few days later, the CFO called again, "Stop by."

I popped by, "What's up?"

"We have offered Miss J the position and she assured us she can pick-up the pieces and successfully manage the entire installation. What a relief."

"Bravo!"

When Senator Robert Kennedy was shot he was first taken to the Central Receiving Emergency Center and from there admitted to our hospital. I had pre-arranged to take the day off (having worked the prior total weekend), so I was away from the office when the senator was transferred to our facility. After listening to the news on the radio, I cancelled my tennis date and other plans and headed to work. There were crowds of people and TV units outside of our main hospital entrance. By the time I arrived, all locations were sealed off except the main entrance.

When I reported for duty, the CFO and administrator agreed that I should take command and station myself at the main entrance reception area to assist the police and others in the screening process. We had a very large medical staff. Fortunately, I knew, or at least could readily identify, every physician who entered the hospital, enabling me to give the high sign to the police. I also helped our volunteers in accompanying family members and other visitors to specific patient rooms. I knew some of our patients and personally accompanied their family and visitors to their rooms. I also assisted in fulfilling requests for the Kennedy aides and other visiting VIPs.

The character actress Mary Wickes, who made her debut playing the nurse in the famous 1940s movie *The Man Who Came to Dinner*, starring Monty Woolley, was also an active volunteer. She was assigned to the reception desk. She, being a down-to-earth lady, helped me by assisting many of the local prominent persons who had stopped by sadly to pay their respects to the Kennedy family and staff.

A visiting physician from Argentina, who had met the senator earlier in Washington, stopped by to try and see the Kennedy family. The police assigned him to me. I spoke with him and took him to a waiting area on a nursing floor.

Taking the initiative, I proceeded to the unit assigned to the Kennedy family. I latched on to a member of the secret service, who responded, "What kind of a Mickey Mouse situation is this? Get him to hell out of here." On second thought, he decided to join me, met the doctor, and requested that he leave immediately.

Television news personalities Roger Mudd and Robert Abernathy were both stationed at the main entrance. Abernathy and I both lived in Pacific Palisades. I had spoken with him briefly after church one Sunday regarding his special weekly program addressed to high school students. It was interesting to note that the actual physicians taking care of the senator were freely walking by both newscasters at the main entrance, but the newsmen didn't realize who they were. I was tempted to give them the high sign for recognition, but realized that that would have been very disingenuous on my part. The entire situation was so very sad for the Kennedy family and those so very close to them.

It was an interesting experience to see all of the family members and friends—Ethel and Ted Kennedy, Jacqueline Kennedy, Patricia Lawford (sister of President Kennedy and wife of actor Peter), and Mrs. Martin Luther King, Jr., who had just shortly before lost her husband. It was an election year and prominent political candidates and representatives from both state and federal governments were at the hospital to pay their respects to the family.

Singer Andy Williams and his wife Claudine Longet were also present. For me, having to experience seeing so many prominent personages at one rather confined area was somewhat overwhelming. I was highly commended for my assigned placatory role during this sad period.

One of the nicest patients I ever worked with was a soft-spoken black lady in her late thirties. She was in charge of an executive dining room for a major bank and became very ill and required surgery and extensive outpatient services. Her insurance paid for her hospitalization in full, but she was required to co-pay for outpatient services. I worked closely with her and arranged to accept insurance only for the outpatient services. I made her promise that she would not worry as I had taken care of any remaining charges. She was extremely grateful and, unfortunately, after a few months she passed away. Her employer called and said she had left the hospital a $2,000 donation from the proceeds of her benefits settlement and that the check was to be delivered personally to me. I cried!

I had been attending classes at UCLA at their downtown location and at their campus while working at both oil companies. While at The Hospital of the Good Samaritan, I decided to take a few classes in marketing. This was the 1960s, and marketing of hospital services was unheard of in the healthcare industry. I felt like an orphan when both the instructor and other students realized that I was in healthcare. I latched on to a couple of pharmaceutical representatives who were taking a series of marketing courses, too. I laughingly joked with them stating, "Treat me as a cousin not an orphan!"

I was just ahead of the crowd, as marketing soon began to play a part in the healthcare industry. I had envisioned the great potential benefits of marketing for healthcare.

I informed our administrative people to look at all of the businesses in the downtown area for potential marketing. Many of their employees were having their services provided in Santa Monica, Long Beach, and other cities, when they could come for treatment and follow-up more accessibly at our hospital. They informed me that my point was well taken but we would never market our services. They said doctors wouldn't advertise their services the same way attorneys would never market their services. They actually thought it was pretty funny.

The 1960s were an unimaginative time. Our UCLA marketing professor requested permission to pilot an advanced special program that would include my pharmaceutical cousins and me. We were all excited, but it fell through at the last minute as he couldn't get funding.

Progressively, later, UCLA designed a special two-year program that covered healthcare, which I attended. It covered all aspects relating to my specific field. I befriended the doctor who was in charge of the program as he was terrific to me and approved one of my program suggestions. In taking vocationally related programs, I had the opportunity to meet others in the industry and to discuss mutual concerns and, in some instances, network together. I tried to incorporate my school projects with my actual work so that both my study and my vocation would benefit—particularly in marketing when it belatedly hit the horizon.

While I was enrolled in that special program, I found a wonderful store on Wilshire Boulevard that sold used books. I used to go there often. They were blessed with a very literate patronage that purchased and exchanged quality books with rapidity. I loved that store and purchased their many treasured books regularly. I picked up one for the doctor who was responsible for the two-year healthcare program. I met him the following week, just before class started. "Dr. M, I was browsing through my favorite bookstore last week and picked up a little gift for you."

"You did? A book I presume?"

"I knew that you had spent sometime in the UK and I found a small but interesting book on Bartholomew Hospital in London."

"Bartholomew Hospital. I spent time there. I can't believe that you found a book on that hospital—and you're giving it to me as a gift."

"How interesting."

"Gus, why didn't you bring it to class tonight?"

"The book is at home and I came directly from work this evening."

"Gus, it's going to be difficult to have to wait for a week to receive my gift. Please put that book in your car when you get home tonight so you don't forget to bring it next week."

"You are so excited, but truthfully it is just a small book, but with quality binding."

He reiteratively said, "I can't wait to receive it, so put it in your car tonight."

I am a gift giver; however, I have never seen anyone demonstrate such appreciation in accepting this small book. He said it was a treasure. It proved the old proverb that it is better to give than to receive. His two-year program at UCLA was excellent and the book was a very small token of my appreciation. I concur with that old adage that the joy of giving is so much more rewarding than the joy of receiving.

12

The executive secretary from Richfield Oil was hospitalized and I made a courtesy visit to see how she was doing. She quite took me by surprise by admonishing me for leaving Richfield Oil, stating I had left a great future. While it was complimentary to me, she did express her thoughts rather unpleasantly.

Prior to this incident, my former manager, Jack, had come for lunch one day, hoping to talk me into returning to Richfield Oil. Before we went to lunch, one of the admitting nurses came rushing into my office stating there was a problem situation at our emergency side entrance. The patient had a drug problem and he kept coming to our facility instead of going to central receiving or the county hospital. I went running to the area with Jack following closely behind. I spoke with the patient and gave the ambulance attendant instructions. They drove off and Jack thought this incident rather exciting. He said, "Are you constantly involved in all of these types of situations?"

I mendaciously said, "Yes!"

He said, "Are you really happy here?"

I said, "Yes!"

Sadly, that was the last time I saw him, as he was convinced I would not be returning to his company. His efforts, too, were most complimentary. Jack apparently accepted a position later with the company in Alaska at the time of all of the exploration and pipeline activity there. By that time, the Richfield Oil Corporation and the Atlantic Refining Company were united to form ARCO. Jack was a great person and unstintingly recognized my work performance and placed me in a very special category. He could be extremely critical—expressively so to those individuals who did not perform to his high standard. In hindsight, I regret having lost touch with him. He had been a mentor and important person in my life. Miraculously, I did survive those frightening joy rides he'd taken me on!

Jack had a good sense of humor and possessed great and strong proficiencies in fulfilling his managerial duties for the organization. Aside from being a rebel in working with the company elite, he was somewhat of a ladies' man.

The year I started with The Hospital of the Good Samaritan, an annual healthcare conference was held in Beverly Hills. It was a national event, and representatives from major hospitals across the country were to attend.

I discussed the conference with my CFO and wondered if the topics discussed would be over my head, as I had been in the field for only a few months. She laughed and said that I would be able to hold my own on all subjects covered. And she was right. In attending that conference and others like it, both nationally and locally, I soon learned that there was a tremendous turnover of persons holding comparable positions to mine in other hospitals.

As I gained more experience and gathered more data, I soon learned that my position in other hospitals was often staffed with incompetent persons. I would attend meetings and listen to my peers discussing job changes all of the time. They were simply moving from one hospital to another. There seemed to be an inordinate amount of volatility related to job performance. Because of this, I never attempted to build relationships with my counterparts in other hospitals. I discouraged any involvement, with the exception of one or two individuals.

When I entered the healthcare field after nine years in the petroleum business, I found accountability to be extremely important. My first day at the hospital, I pulled trays of accounts into my office to review for completeness and activity. The CFO was delighted observing my immediate involvement in our accounts receivable and made laudatory comments.

I immediately, strengthened our follow-up systems, developed a series of letters, and initiated other useful collection tools. Actually, I learned that, for a large hospital, we were in good shape and that our systems and employees were great. I worked continuously on our accounts and all financial situations and monitored them appropriately. I still had time to develop good working relationships with our patients and their family members—and, additionally, with all departments and, importantly, with our medical staff and their personnel.

In another area of accountability, I approved the release of valuables to a family member, after the death of a loved one at our hospital. One time, this transaction caused another family member to complain vociferously. The CFO and I met with nursing administration over this potential debacle, and, during our meeting, I decided to call the coroner's office and review the issue step by step. It turned out to be a very lengthy telephone conversation. Being a novice in this type of situation, I just simply pleaded guilty for any wrongdoing and took full responsibility. When hearing the total situation, the representative at the coroner's office stated that I had acted in good faith and no wrongdoing was involved. She actually supported me completely, stating my actions in that situation had been appropriate. All of the administrative top brass attended this meeting and they were delighted that the situation was verifiably resolved amicably.

Returning to our office, the CFO said, "Mr. Munro, you are unquestionably a man of honor, placing yourself in what could have been an untenable position. Your integrity showed above everything else and I was beaming with pride during your entire performance. You just simply and clearly laid it on the line in accepting responsibility."

"Thanks for your kind words; however, a lesson was to be learned in addressing those specific issues. And I don't take that lesson lightly. That lady at the coroner's office will be a good resource for me when addressing future similar issues."

One of our most prominent physicians actually occupied one part of a third-floor wing exclusively for his patients, along with a small office. By the time we met, he was an elderly gentleman who had apparently mellowed over the years. However, according to nursing administration, he was still demanding and quite contentious. When he needed me to discuss one of his patients, we would meet in his hospital office. Invariably, he would be relaxed and he would nod off momentarily and then awaken and resume his conversation exactly where he had left off. I must interject parenthetically that he was a medical doctor only—he did not do any surgeries. For some unknown reason, he took a liking to me and he was always extremely affable during our discussions.

One day he met me at the main entrance and shook my hand and informed me I did a wonderful job at the hospital. He said he needed to shake my hand every time we met. He had a luxurious town car, complete with chauffeur, and one day he spotted me near the Farmers Market. He had his chauffeur stop the car so he could greet me and to ask if I needed a lift. I didn't, but I loved the VIP treatment.

I worked closely with one of the nursing administrators and she couldn't believe how courteous this doctor was to me. She said he was an excellent physician and great with his patients, but a hellion to work with. She went on to say that I had certainly been privileged. I dismissed any negative comments, as he was very special to me.

His name has prominently been mentioned in many Hollywood biographies. He took care of so many celebrities over the years, including the gorgeous, but tragic, Jean Harlow, who expired so young at our hospital.

It was not unusual to pass many of the older movie stars in the hallways that were at our hospital for medical services. One day, looking out of my office window, I saw an older woman—not beautiful but with pronounced stature and grace in her walk. I assumed she was someone of importance. She turned out to be the legendary Canadian actress, Norma Shearer, who was hospitalized but ambulatory. She seemed to epitomize by grace and stature the 1930s image of the glamorous Hollywood actress. However, her poise and movement appeared to me quite staged.

One of the most stunningly beautiful older actresses was Gail Patrick, who played secondary movie roles in the 1930s and '40s. For many years in television she was the executive producer of the *Perry Mason* series as Gail Patrick Jackson. She and Rosemary were having an in-depth conversation in the admitting office one afternoon and I joined them. Later, Rosemary commented that she thought Gail Patrick Jackson was a very bright businesswoman. I was incredibly captivated by her ageless beauty.

We would see other old-time stars such as John Wayne, Randolph Scott, Frank Sinatra, and Katherine Hepburn, along with designer Edith Head and many TV personalities passing through our admitting department and main lobby.

I had the pleasure of meeting a prominent producer who had been with MGM Studios for many years. He was a patient and a very affable and interesting person. He mentioned that he had worked with all of the important stars at that studio and commented favorably on many. He informed me that I was, as they say, professionally handsome and mentioned a possible screen test.

He was very complimentary in his comments; however, I let it pass as I hated reading aloud in front of others. When attending meetings and educational workshops, I dreaded having to stand and read unfamiliar material without preparation and advanced reading.

I was grateful when the Medicare program came into effect on July 1, 1966. We had so many older patients who had pre-existing conditions that prevented them from having private insurance coverage and/or had conditions that were excluded from their policies. Many of these patients had been drained of their financial resources because of these insurance restrictions. I spent a lot of time assisting our patients in learning about Medicare—it seemed so complex with deductibles and other stipulations. I worked very closely in providing Medi-Cal (indigent care program) services to our patients, particularly through our clinical services, and I was instrumental in contacting the state of California on issues relating to Share of Cost and other coverage.

In the infancy of Medi-Cal I would address issues with the state that were not clearly defined. They actually appreciated my intervention and input, particularly relating to the patient share of cost and other coverage issues. It was a learning process at both the state level and hospital level. Based on my own personal experience, our combined input and cooperation was jointly and greatly appreciated in addressing any anomalies.

In being responsible for our patient accounts, I spent a great deal of my time auditing accounts receivable for payment. I also reviewed the timeliness of billing and follow-up procedures. Fortunately, we had quality personnel and I was able to expand my roles in other areas that were more beneficial to our patients and the hospital. It was one hospital where I didn't need to spend many hours a week monitoring our accounts receivable.

While at The Hospital of the Good Samaritan, I realized that I needed some professional help in my personal life. In many quarters, and even as close as some members of our administrative staff, the thought of contemplating seeking medical assistance for emotional conditions was frowned upon. I surreptitiously found a great psychiatrist in West Los Angeles and started treatment with him. Apart from knowing that I did have insurance benefits to cover treatment, I fully realized that my problems related to my parents, childhood, dropping out of school, and loving but not liking my wife.

I informed the doctor that I personally would pay for treatment as I went along. I had no intention of charging the hospital, through their insurance plan, for problems that were unrelated to work. My doctor was wonderful. I would periodically stop treatment to financially bring myself up to date, and then I would resume treatment again.

Being a physician, he was astutely aware that I had a responsible position at the hospital. He occasionally mentioned that I never ever had the need to discuss work issues with him.

I always responded that I understood my work. I definitely had no conflict regarding all of the ramifications in managing multiple departments or working out employee problems. I would periodically mention a human-interest story relating to a member of my staff and tell him how I addressed the situation. He actually gave me high marks and informed me that I was very in tune in addressing employee problems and their concerns. My doctor informed me that he was impressed with my astuteness and insight into his field; he even suggested that I go back to school and become a psychologist. I declined that suggestion; I felt it was a little too late to start. His suggestion did encourage me to discuss many employee problems that had been brought to my attention. Talking them out often helped me to solve them.

Almost immediately in starting treatment, he informed me that I displayed excessive compulsive behavior. I was able to quickly discern how the rigidity that is a signpost of this disorder was affecting my life and the way I was facing my problems.

Essentially, I was turning my anger inward instead of addressing a problem and seeking a solution. I seemed to be able to identify other persons' problems and help to resolve them, but I kept my own problems in a repetitious state of confusion or limbo. The doctor helped me to better understand my compulsive behavior—wanting everything orderly and seeking perfectionism at both work and home. I paradoxically, during thoughtful moments, realized that this condition had been the cause of my constant frustration with my father and the poker and party crowd. His lifestyle and mine could never have existed together in harmonious accord.

My sister Laura passed away very suddenly at the age of forty-one. She was truly the most beautiful woman I have ever known, and that assessment has been echoed by most of the persons who had known her. She was about five foot six, always very slim and chic, and looked like a fashion model, but not as willowy. She had long, thick sleekly jet black hair and dark brown sparkling eyes, great proportional features, and a flawlessly clear, very white complexion that contrasted strikingly with her dark hair.

In appearance she was between Ava Gardener and Ann Miller. I had seen Ann Miller up close and had seen a resemblance. While no Ann Miller, Laura was a great dancer—both tap and ballroom dancing—and I believe she possessed great undeveloped potentialities in that field. During the depression years, Laura's talent was so promising that her teacher included her in classes and simply waived her fees.

Certain promises were made to her in her earlier years in the direction of Hollywood; however, nothing was formulated and nothing materialized. I always questioned the motives of those in her circle who were simply on the fringe of show business. During the era of nightclub entertainment, many of our Canadian or visiting American show-biz characters would make false assertions to attractive women as a ploy to feed their sybaritic lifestyles. Laura was always taken in.

While my father, sister Marjorie and I were still together in the earlier years, Laura would occasionally return home for brief periods. She, too, was a neat freak and, on one occasion, returned home and spent the entire night creatively rearranging our living room, scouring our bathroom and kitchen, and washing and waxing floors and furniture. She actually crawled right into the bathtub to clean it. She completed this project at close to 5:00 AM and excitedly got us all up just to admire her work. For me, her visits were too infrequent.

Laura was a tremendous self-trained pastry chef and would bake a variety of pies and other goodies on any given day. Years later, during one of her productive periods, she worked as a pastry chef at one of the most prestigious hotels in Canada, which was no surprise to me. However, her productive periods were short lived, as her emotional demonic tendencies would resurface to take her down the negative path once more, seemingly a never-ending repetitious cycle.

At the time of her death, she was in a relationship with a prosperous fisherman who owned and operated a large fishing vessel between Vancouver and Prince Rupert.

I learned that Laura and some friends had just returned from the annual Calgary Stampede and she met her mate in Prince Rupert. From there, they spent time along the coastal waters for a couple of days. Apparently, during the return period on the boat, her mate noticed that she was extremely happy, effervescent, and lighthearted. However, suddenly she died one evening soon afterwards in her sleep. I have heard that this type of pre-death behavior is not uncommon.

My sister Marjorie and I returned to Vancouver after hearing the news. Laura's body was returned to Vancouver, accompanied by her mate. We met with him and several of Laura's friends at the Mount Pleasant Funeral Parlour. I was actually surprised to see all of her friends there ahead of the funeral as I, accompanied by my sister and mother, were there solely to make the funeral service arrangements.

Laura's mate was extremely well mannered, very courteous, and visually ravaged with sadness and disbelief over her sudden passing. The other men and women who were present were also shocked and deeply moved. My sister Laura, unless annoyed at me, always called me, "Angie" as a form of endearment. While she was constant in addressing me as such, no friend or family member ever called me by that special nickname. The women present, whom I had never met previously, were calling me by her name for me, too. While it appeared strange to me, they must have assumed that it was my accepted nickname. However, in deference, I said nothing. I was actually somewhat moved by their familiarity, assuming, just from my observations, that Laura must have conveyed a favorable picture of me to them.

Needless to say, this was very somber gathering. However, even through his tears, Laura's mate brought forth some humor. Apparently, Laura's trip to the Calgary Stampede was a spur-of-the-moment decision, and I assumed she had left Prince Rupert to meet friends in Vancouver to join her and carry on to Calgary. During the mate's absence, she had taken funds from his cash box to cover the trip. When she returned from Calgary, her mate confronted her and said, "You took over one thousand dollars out of the cash box."

She said, "I did not. It was only eight hundred dollars." Everyone roared with laughter, and the mate was tearfully laughing too.

Despite the sadness, I felt so much better meeting her mate and wonderful friends. Laura was so special to me—so beautiful, so gifted and so abused with turmoil throughout her short life. It was all so regrettable and incomprehensible.

Unfortunately, her proclivities and attractions to men with nefarious backgrounds were contributors to her downfall. Over the years, she became involved with drugs and all that is associated with that lifestyle including the heavy financial demands of maintaining that negative habit. Not being very street-smart, I can only surmise she was plagued by an involvement with theft, prostitution, and incarceration, followed by rehabilitation and ongoing relationships with male users and cheaters. I recall seeing her in Vancouver on one of my trips. During that period she was living a more constructive lifestyle. I posed the question, "In working through rehabilitation with your therapist, have you received any insight that might help you understand your current lifestyle?"

She simply said, "My therapist informed me that I hated my mother." Unfortunately, she never ever worked through it, but, instead, focused on her own negative, guilt-ridden lifestyle. She suppressed the reality of the original cause of her unhappiness and followed a lifetime of pain and suffering.

Laura had a lifetime of ups and downs, sorrow and anguish. Onlookers in those days—the 1940s and '50s—were unsophisticated and we addressed negative behavior with one-liners rather than working to find the underlying causes or demonstrating compassion. I must confess that I was originally one who delivered those one-liners, a fact that later riddled me with sorrow, anger, and shame; however, my wonderful therapist introduced me to reality—a somewhat rocky road to travel, but the destination is all that truly matters. Seek and you shall find. When you reach the top of the hill you look down and all of the parts of your seemingly disjointed journey fit like a completed Mrs. Giggle-Britches puzzle. Eureka!

On a parting note, Laura had the most wonderful sense of humor. I have used some of her material over the years very effectively when making presentations. She and I both particularly loved children's comments that are so simply stated without any intention of being humorous. She actually overheard an exchange between two five-year-old lads: One lad was showing off his new shoes to the other. The other lad replied, "You are so lucky. I have had these old shoes for about ten years!"

Laura had been exposed to many interesting people in her life—from all walks of life—but she always said that my humor was unparalleled. This was probably an overstatement, but our joint humor served to suppress our joint sadness in early childhood events. We shared a special bond that was loaded with suppression and unresolved issues.

Upon my return from Vancouver, one morning, one of my cashiers came charging into my office to discuss a personal concern. "Mr. Munro, I am madly in love with you and I am getting a bottle of champagne and I am going to tell the world how I feel about you."

"I suggest you sit down and let's quietly discuss this situation."

"There is nothing to discuss! I cannot continue hiding my feelings for you."

"It is my understanding that you have had some problems at home with visitation issues regarding your parents and your husband's parents?"

"Yes, first his parents stayed for a prolonged period. Finally, I asked my husband to tell them to leave. They would have stayed forever."

"Shortly thereafter, your parents arrived and they, too, stayed for a prolonged period before they finally left."

"Yes, that is true."

"I believe that you are conveniently using me as a scapegoat. You feel guilty because you evicted his parents. Your husband, conversely, did not oppose the fact that your parents stayed just as long."

"Mr. Munro, you are right about both sets of parents—and especially my hostile reaction to his parents being there so long."

"Trust me when I tell you that you are not madly in love with me. You are conveniently using me as a cover up to your true feelings. It is called displacement."

"I know how I feel about you."

"This is what I want you to do. This evening, sit down and talk with your husband regarding the visits of both parents. Tell him that you are feeling very guilty over the fact that you gave his parents the bum's rush, while he silently accepted the fact that your parents remained for a long period, too."

"I don't understand all of this, but I need to talk to him because I do feel guilty as you suggest."

"Trust me, I believe you love your husband and essentially have a good marriage."

Two or three weeks later she returned to my office, "Mr. Munro, thank you for your help. You were right. I really felt guilty and I got my feelings completely screwed up. My husband and I are now doing well, thanks to your good advice."

Closing thoughts—dumped but delighted! My doctor loved this story.

The nephew of one of our top brass came to work part-time in our department. He had just completed college and planned to work full-time during the summer and return to college in the fall to work on his master's program. He planned to work part-time thereafter. He worked in the cashiers unit and I worked every Saturday and occasionally on Sundays performing audits or follow-ups, or on special projects. He immediately volunteered his services over the weekends during the lull periods. He could type well and he sent out letters or notices to patients for me. His work was excellent and he was diligent. He also was lots of fun and had a good sense of humor, but he got the job done.

He would volunteer to run out at lunchtime on the weekends and pick-up something different from a restaurant or a fast food joint. We really enjoyed having him around as he balanced his humor with hard work.

One Saturday while another cashier was also on duty, he took some work from me and started to take it to the next office. Suddenly, but quietly, he said he had something to tell me, "I wish you were my father." he said.

I took his comments very lightly and said, "Gosh, I was just nineteen-years-old when you were born!" Then I got more serious, "Come on, tell me about your father and your relationship with him, and let's try and discern the real problem."

I befriended him, went to his graduation at UCLA with his family, and accepted an invitation for dinner at his home with his parents and brother and sister. They were truly a nice family, and they had worked hard to purchase a new home.

His father had recently changed jobs and acquired a more elevated position and he was feeling more personally challenged. The father, I believe, had felt inferior to his siblings over their scholastic success, and his new position gave him an impetus to fulfill new goals and broaden his horizon. My new young friend's brother and sister were both in college and extremely bright and performing well. Certainly raising three successful children should be a credit to both parents. We continued to work together and we had a very special bond. He eventually became an engineer and he and his father seemed to develop a better rapport. My assessment was that they were a very close, productive, and caring family.

13

While we lived in Los Angeles, my wife and I decided to move nearer to the ocean. We met a lady and her husband who owned four units in Santa Monica a few blocks from the cliffs, overlooking the beach and the Pacific Ocean. Their front units were an irregular duplex—the owners' unit being somewhat larger than the rental unit, which became ours. They also owned two additional rental units in back, which were constructed above the four-car garage. The husband had worked for a governmental agency and he passed away not too long after we moved into their complex.

Our landlady Maybelle was retired, but had been very entrepreneurial. She had owned a dress shop and she was also a milliner by vocation. She had conducted both businesses simultaneously and adroitly. As a milliner, she would visit her clients in their homes. One of her clients had been former screen star Marion Davies, and Maybelle had visited her at her famous beach home. (Marion Davies was the partner to newspaper tycoon William Randolph Hearst.)

Maybelle absolutely adored my wife and made her some beautiful dresses. My wife had a model's figure that complemented Maybelle's dressmaking skills. My wife was really delighted and so appreciative.

Aside from being extremely talented, Maybelle told interesting stories about the older Hollywood stars—a mix from the silent era and "talkies," too.

After we had resided with her for about four years we purchased a small home in the Pacific Palisades. She came to dinner one evening. At the dinner table, she informed my wife and me that she was going to paint a picture just like the one in her living room.

The picture was of a lion overlooking the ocean, which to me appeared both fatuous and grotesque with an underlining bizarreness. This was strange, as she normally had impeccable taste in all aspects. The picture was truly dreadful. My wife said, "Oh no, Gus doesn't like that picture."

Maybelle was taken back by her comments, and I was ready to crawl under the table. After we drove her home, I asked my wife why she had made those comments about me regarding the picture, even though I agreed that it was awful. She laughingly said, "I hate that picture, what else could I say?" Her comment had been funny, but very embarrassing, and I had been rendered speechless at the time. But we laughed all the way home.

Maybelle had been a great friend for almost a dozen years, and then a horrible tragedy occurred. She used an electric blanket, and one evening it shorted and she inhaled the simmering smoke. The smoke killed her before the conflagration broke out that destroyed her bedroom floor. Her bed looked like a burned tomb. After the fire, the bedroom and remnants were dreadful and macabre. She had an elderly sister who was an artist and a wonderful lady, who, needless to say, was totally distraught after the horrible incident. She, at the time, was residing in one of Maybelle's back units.

The sister eventually had a sale of Maybelle's fine china, crystal, furniture, and artwork, and she asked that I select anything I wanted before the sale began. She said, "Whatever you want, take."

I replied, "Thank you, but everything I need is in my heart. I need nothing more."

At the hospital I worked very closely in addressing patient concerns regarding insurance coverage and benefits relating to our ancillary departments, such as physical therapy, occupational therapy, and radiation therapy. While I worked closely with the department heads of outpatient services, I particularly worked almost daily with the chief radiologist in radiation therapy. He would insist that every single patient see me and he was totally hands-on in addressing their needs, both medical and financial. I would personally get verifications of coverage on their insurance and keep the doctor apprised on everything. I developed a good rapport with his patients and he received many favorable comments about me. He wanted to be certain that no patient (even those with full benefit coverage) was excluded from my personal intervention. He was a tough taskmaster and demanding in addressing the needs of his patients. I frankly admired his work ethic.

Personally, I believe both he and his wife were old movie buffs, and he would tell me where many of the old classic movies had been made on location outside of the studios in the LA area. It was interesting to hear about the locations and events, especially as I am an old movie buff, too. These tales were also a welcomed temporary diversion from difficult patient issues. I personally admired his professionalism and unstinting dedication to his patients. He was a remarkable human being, but he was demanding and a handful to work with. Through it all we had a great rapport, as he knew my standards were high, too.

When I first started working with radiation therapy patients, I met a young lady and a young man, unknown to each other and both younger than I. They were very attractive and looked great, but apparently their prognoses were not too encouraging. When either one left my office, I became tearfully remorseful in trying to cope with their plight. I surreptitiously developed a kinship toward both of them, but conducted my conversations in a friendly but businesslike manner. I was totally ill equipped and emotionally weak in accepting their illnesses. It seemed so tragic and incomprehensible because both were so young. I included them in my daily prayers. However, in terms of assisting these patients with their insurance and related issues, I did everything possible to help them. That was my contribution—befittingly to help in any way.

I found it difficult to work with terminally ill patients; however, I eventually found help when I attended a conference that featured Dr. Elisabeth Kubler-Ross as guest speaker. I attended the meeting as I had heard that this woman was incredibly outstanding. She seemed to address her speech to each single individual in attendance. It was a phenomenal experience—and inexplicable.

Dr. Kubler-Ross was a Swiss physician who devoted her practice to death and dying. Indeed, her famous book is titled *Death and Dying*. Her lectures were inspirational in addressing the needs of terminally ill patients.

On a much lighter note, one of the assistant nursing office directors, Agnes, who was nearing sixty years old, shared an apartment with her sister, who was about two years her senior. They were both spinsters and their apartment was on Wilshire Boulevard and near the hospital. They had resided there for many years.

Nursing salaries were not very high, and practicing frugality was necessary. While Agnes had a good position, to augment her salary she did private-duty nursing after hours. Her patient was the wife of a president of one of the largest and most prestigious law firms in the United States, which was headquartered in Los Angeles.

After a prolonged illness, the patient died. Her husband became smitten with Agnes and they married when Agnes had just reached sixty. This marriage certainly opened new doors for her. She quickly adjusted to her new lifestyle, as she was a very refined and gregarious lady to begin with—as was her sister.

Upon marriage, they introduced the sister to an unattached and very wealthy man in Beverly Hills, and they, too, were married shortly thereafter. Those two sisters, who had lived very quiet and frugal lives, suddenly became extremely wealthy and socially very prominent. Their lives flowed graciously with these events. They retained their nursing colleagues and other associates at the hospital—inviting them to many of their parties and other social functions.

Agnes's husband stopped by my office one day for a brief chat. He had the "poor me" syndrome, stating grudgingly that his wife had put him on a very strict diet. I jokingly said, "It's your fault—you married a nurse and all that healthy stuff goes with it!"

He laughingly responded, "I must confess—you're right, Gus!"

For a very prominent LA executive, he was down to earth and treated his wife's former hospital associates in a very dignifying and friendly manner. One would have never predicted that those two little gals would receive such happiness and opulence in their later years. In appearance they were certainly the antitheses of the glamorous Gabor sisters—but they made it up by circumstance.

Being near Santa Monica, a tennis community, I took some tennis lessons from an instructor who was working at the Lincoln Tennis Courts, a few blocks up from the beach. My instructor mentioned that he had another student who was an executive with KLM Dutch Airlines, who wanted to meet me for tennis. So, I met Carlos. He was ten years my senior and extremely bright. He spoke five languages fluently. He was from Spain and was married (his second marriage) to a former flight attendant who was American, and a gorgeous lady. He was very European, had excellent manners, was articulate and immaculately groomed. He had a tremendous sense of humor. He had been raised in Spain as a member of a prominent upper-class family—what seemed to me just a step below Spanish nobility.

He had received his higher education in England. One of his classmates was the politician John Profumo, who later married the English actress Valerie Hobson. (Profumo was involved in the infamous sex scandal involving Christine Keeler and some British spies who were involved with the Soviets—it was a mess!) Carlos had spent his summers in France as a child. He spoke English, Spanish, French, Italian, and German. He showed no trace of elitism; he was engagingly and humorously down to earth.

One day Carlos was speaking German to a young lady on the tennis court. As their conversation was incessant, he sounded commandingly fluent, but he told me that German was his worst language. Further, he said that his linguistic skills were less than those of his brother, who was a linguist with the United Nations and spoke one or two more languages than he. For a brilliant man, he spoke very simplistically and laconically about himself. I enjoyed his humor and he loved teasing me. Normally, his political conversation was of a higher level than I was used to, and often it was controversial. I found that to be enriching to my thought processes on a variety of topics.

In his youth, Carlos lived in Spain under the Franco regime that had a kinship with Nazi Germany and Italy. His father was a Spanish diplomat and took Carlos on a trip to Germany. At a diplomatic dinner, escorted by their Spanish ambassador, they met both Dr. Josef Goebbels and Adolf Hitler. Carlos stated that Franco was very adroit in remaining out of World War II as part of the Axis pact. He said that Hitler and Franco met by train in Northern Spain and Franco stated the toll of the Spanish Civil War made it unthinkable for Spain to join their camp, as he had his hands full averting any possible internal insurgency. Franco played them all very cunningly and sagaciously and the aftermath was in his favor.

Our friendship came about in the late 1960s, and the fear of the cold war was still running through our veins. Carlos informed me that there would be no war with the then Soviet Union. He envisioned the eventual transformation to Russia with the reunification of Germany and autonomy for the Eastern Block nations.

Carlos also accurately predicted that Europe would soon be economically united, including Russia and all of the Eastern Block nations. He said they would all be capitalistic with a socialistic theme—his prognostications were on target. At the time, it sounded like a platitudinous view and certainly not feasible in my lifetime.

One of Carlos' mother's close friends was the heiress Barbara Hutton. During the 1940s she was married to Cary Grant, and Carlos stayed at their Beverly Hills home on one of his trips to America. He certainly learned the Hollywood tidbits and shared them with us years later. At the time, some of his comments were surprising.

One morning at the Lincoln Courts a man and woman were really having a tremendous workout on the next court. I was to have a lesson after playing with Carlos, and I informed my instructor that I thought I should just go home. He said, "Why?"

I replied, "There is a little gal on the next court hitting the ball like a bullet. She is phenomenal!"

"Gus," said he, "that is the tennis star, Gussie Moran!"

I said, "The famous, gorgeous Gussie "Fancy Pants" Moran?"

"Yeah!" said he.

She had a unique dress style that included ruffle-seated tennis panties. She was famous for wearing them on the tennis courts at Wimbledon, and in the United States, and elsewhere. We started our lesson and the next thing I knew Carlos, along with Gussie and her partner, were watching me. Fortunately, they left soon after, but Carlos remained and conveniently during my session called me over to hand me Gussie's card and telephone number. He said, "She called me over and wanted to meet you and arrange a date for the four of us to play tennis." He excitedly added, "She is really interested in meeting you." I never called her.

Carlos and his wife eventually returned to Spain and settled in Malaga. He offered me a position with the organization that he was going to administer. His firm represented several large holiday and residential complexes and involved wealthy investors from Germany and other countries. I thought it would be a wonderful adventure; however, I rejected his proposal, as I had no bilingual skills. He countered by saying I had good business acumen and I would learn the language quite easily. He was a good friend, a great linguist, and he approached each subject in a very mundane fashion. One of my family members thought he was both contentious and arrogant. He was just assertively expressing his point of view. He told my family I was missing a great opportunity by not moving to Spain.

One of our prominent physicians on staff, Dr. Marinacci, was described as having a pioneering role in the fields of the electroencephalogram (EEG) and the electromyogram (EMG). He was the author of studies in both procedures. He was known for his brilliance, but he unfortunately wore a toupee that appeared to have been designed after Davy Crockett's coonskin cap—not flattering for this near genius. His technical and secretarial services support assistant was an Irish "gal Friday" Teresa who was opinionated but lovable—late forties, honest, straightforward, and a shoot-from-the hip person. With her accent and quick wittedness, she was readily identified as coming from "the Old Sod." She was a wonderful person and totally devoted to her physician. In the hallways, cafeteria, and throughout the hospital, she was always near his side to fulfill any request. She suddenly took ill and was hospitalized at Good Samaritan.

She called me from her hospital room and stated that after two days they were still trying to determine her medical problem. As she carefully and methodically described her symptoms in detail to me, I without thinking said, "It sounds like a gallbladder condition."

"Gus, don't tell me that. My gallbladder?"

"Teresa, forgive me for my stupid comment, I am no doctor—how the hell would I know?"

The day following, Teresa had surgery to remove her gallbladder.

I told this story to one of my physician friends and joshingly asked, "Could they send me up the river for attempted malpractice?"

He facetiously responded, "Did you put that information on the patient's chart or charge for your services?"

"No, I did not!"

Said he, "You are off the hook, but heed this lesson, Gus!"

Teresa's closing comment after her recovery, "Gus, I am impressed. You should have become a doctor!"

After nine successful years at The Hospital of the Good Samaritan I decided to leave. I contemplated the feasibility of moving out of the Los Angeles area. When I informed the CFO (who had formerly been the assistant CFO) she actually started to cry, and I left her office. I spoke with a nursing administrator who said, "I have a little story to tell you."

The hospital was going to select their most outstanding employee and physician. She named the doctor and the employee—Gus Munro. She said the committee said,

"Who could possibly compete with him?" That was a nice send-off for me. It had been a tremendous experience entering the healthcare industry and being associated with such a fine institution.

When the radiologist learned of my pending departure, he unhappily exclaimed, "So you have made yourself indispensable and now you are leaving and telling us all where to go?" as he lifted his right hand and middle finger, making the gesture.

"Sorry about that; time to leave."

"I assume you want a letter from me discussing your attributes in glowing terms?"

"That would be nice." He wrote a wonderful letter. I was told that he informed my replacement soon after he assumed my responsibilities that he was no Gus Munro!

While I was at the hospital, my wife and I, as I mentioned earlier, had purchased a small three-bedroom home in the Pacific Palisades. My wife had been working with a real estate saleslady who was a first cousin to actress Gene Tierney. They looked more like sisters, the resemblance was so strong. While I was still at The Hospital of the Good Samaritan, my wife and I divorced and I sold the home—actually for less than I had paid for it. At the time of the sale there had been a slump in the real estate market, but the same saleslady did her best in selling the property for me.

That was a difficult period in my life as I truly loved my wife but did not like her, which made our situation completely hopeless. When we had first met, we shared a great love affair, but it hadn't lasted very long. We shared the same moral standards, but our personalities clashed. I believe we both tried in vain hoping the situation would change, but it didn't. We didn't play any fault games; we never played the "you did this and I did that" scenario. We were both much better off when we finally parted. Apart from the hollowness of our relationship, she truthfully remains the love of my life—my one-and-only.

When I started at The Hospital of the Good Samaritan in June 1964 my salary was $650 per month, which was considered very good at that time.

I recall that the rates at our prestigious hospital were $33 per day for a private room and $31 per day for a semi-private room. The advent of the Medicare and Medicaid programs in July 1966 provided accessibility to healthcare for special-need categories: seniors who had been unable to afford coverage, or had pre-existing conditions that had been excluded from coverage; and indigent patients, who were, in 1966, afforded coverage through the Medicaid program (Medi-Cal in California).

Hospital facilities, both large and small, grew tremendously to accommodate the new programs. With the increase in patient care, these facilities required more expertise in the management of the programs with their ongoing regulations and requirements. Many smaller hospitals were actually doubling their size under one major expansion project. Salaries in healthcare rose rapidly, along with the need for more nursing and technical services, patient care personnel, medical technology, computerization, and management expertise. Each year at budget time, hospitals were simply increasing their rates to accommodate the financial demands necessary to accommodate expansion of services and increased salaries.

Eventually, retrenchment set in with the introduction of managed care and vast reductions in the Medicare and Medicaid programs through payment based on diagnosis-related groups (DRGs) and other methodologies.

Before I departed The Hospital of the Good Samaritan, a long-term member of my billing staff married a very dynamic executive. It was a second marriage for both.

The husband would often stop by and say hello to me when picking up his wife after work. They had also invited some of our group to their home for parties. When he learned of my pending departure, he and his wife arranged a dinner for me at his country club.

He recently had changed positions and had received a generous package based on his excellent reputation within his industry. At dinner, he informed me that he had witnessed how effectively I had managed my areas of responsibility in the hospital. He also cited how favorably my co-workers had accepted me. He suggested I needed to include those attributes in the negotiating process with a new employer. He was very complimentary and in his words I sensed a strong element of truth. Unfortunately, I did not heed his advice and I really shortchanged myself on numerous occasions. He was very pragmatic and would not have arranged this special dinner totally at his cost unless he felt strongly regarding my performance at the hospital and my overall potential. He was a workaholic, too, extremely effective, and he was reimbursed commensurately.

I had spent nine wonderful years at The Hospital of the Good Samaritan. I truly believe that I found my true self there in terms of responsibilities and interacting so closely with persons and families in need. I loved working with all departments, along with our wonderful medical staff and the administration. It had been an exciting experience being involved in so many projects with so many people. The position had provided total personal fulfillment.

Because the hospital was so prestigious, I had been afforded the opportunity to meet many prominent persons in banking, brokerage houses, retailing, the film industry, manufacturing, the food service industry, and so on. I would never have met these people in my private life. Our conversations were based on their individual needs, or the needs of others, and they were seeking my advice and assistance. My assistance in addressing issues with both patients and/or their representatives always seemed to be accepted with alacrity.

We discussed issues, approaches, and compromises very amicably—and considered each other as equals. These were very engaging exchanges and I sorely needed them to uplift my inner feeling of inadequacy and self-doubt. Quite frankly, I received numerous compliments, and one prominent banker stopped one of my co-workers and said, "What does Mr. Munro prefer to drink socially?"

"He loves gin and tonic."

"What? With a name like Angus Munro, he should be drinking scotch!" And I received scotch from him as a gift. My wife's brother was visiting us and he loved every drop.

I am not a social climber; however, I find it interesting to meet people from all walks of life. We are all here on this earth, taking our individual paths and experiencing good and bad periods, dealing and accepting what is dealt to us. And our visits here maybe long or short as we all face the same commonality; namely, the unknown.

While I sadly said farewell, I was really excited, as I had accepted a position as manager of patient accounts at St. John's Regional Medical Center in Oxnard, California. The Oxnard/Ventura area was a small, quiet community and I was really happy to be situated in a semi-rural atmosphere. My managerial duties included the inpatient and outpatient admitting units and the business office. The staffing complement for these units was fifty-five persons. I also knew that Ventura County would be great for my personal activities—tennis, golfing, hiking, track, speed walking, not to mention the beach and ocean-fresh air.

14

When I started at St. John's Regional Medical Center (SJRMC), I quickly realized that my role there would be far more demanding and challenging than it had
been at The Hospital of the Good Samaritan. I was now in charge of the admitting office and patient representatives, the emergency room registration and outpatient services admitting units as well as the business office. At The Hospital of
the Good Samaritan my primary focus and base had been in business services and
working with the other units as a secondary slot. I had been constantly involved
with many departments and physician-related issues at Good Samaritan, working
with administrative colleagues and others in the decision-making process. At
SJRMC, I quickly felt more "in the trenches." I was totally responsible for the
admitting areas as well.

In hindsight, based on my limited time at SJRMC, the best decision I made
when entering the healthcare field was not accepting that first position offered to
me at the other very large and prestigious hospital. I would have been totally
unequipped in accepting such a challenging position as an initial entry. Good
Samaritan had defined procedures and offered no emergency room services,
which eliminated a tremendous amount of time and effort.

Good Samaritan had an established clinical program, staffed with social workers to provide services for both child and adult indigent care. All of their functions and procedures were handled through the charity services at their Good
Hope Clinic. All patients had insurance and/or the funds to cover their hospital
costs or were under the (prescreened) Good Hope Program. Working with those
established programs afforded me the opportunity to learn all of the rudimentary
and advanced aspects through my personal involvement. While I addressed
important issues, I did not do so in a crisis mode. Time was normally available to
methodically work through each new challenge or opportunity. Yes, anomalies
occurred, but in a calmer environment.

When you work only at one hospital you have no idea what exists in other
places. When starting at SJRMC, I realized the benefits of the experience and
observations I had experienced while working at Good Samaritan. Yes, I came
well versed and prepared for the challenges at this new hospital. I continually
compared one hospital to the other. At Good Samaritan, for example, our admit-

ting office had been staffed with nurses (registered nurses or licensed vocational nurses), and at SJRMC the admitting office was staffed with lay personnel only. I was used to speaking with trained medical personnel, and at SJRMC our admitting representatives had no medical background. I learned that the latter was the most common in the hospital field. Thus, I learned new enlightenments by observation.

Before my arrival at SJRMC, the hospital had undergone some information systems changes. To further accommodate the business office, a methods and procedures specialist had worked with the business office, restructuring it from beginning to end.

I had a background of order and simplicity. I soon changed many impractical and/or redundant procedures that had been set in place by the specialist. My staff welcomed the practicality of those changes. I soon learned that I was having ongoing meetings with various units in my departments—most were initiated by my disgruntled staff.

It all seemed a chaotic mess and I soon learned that we could not be running around all day to unproductive meetings and not getting the work done and problems solved. At Good Samaritan we had had a staffing complement of persons who had longevity of employment. I had expected the same at SJRMC as it was located in a smaller and seemingly more stable community. Contrary to my assumption, the staffing pattern was very unstable and erratic, which was a real concern to me as I cherish stability and consistency. My plan was simply to fix one thing at a time and move on to the next.

The billing supervisor was a very vivacious, attractive lady who dressed tastefully. She was a "people person" and not one to be burdened with the pressures of keeping the billing department current and addressing all of the related internal and external requirements—that simply was not her forte. At the first opportunity, I transferred her to our patient representative unit, relieving her of the pressure. Her personality enhanced her new unit and the staff and public all welcomed her. I promoted a very knowledgeable, diligent and prolific billing specialist to succeed her. Each move was beneficial to each department. I made other internal changes as we progressed step by step.

One area badly needing assistance was outpatient billing. My first Saturday at work, I observed that they had a full staff working on the billing backlog and I sensed a tremendous amount of negativity. I arrived very early the following Saturday and jumped right in by grabbing a handful of accounts that needed to be billed. The outpatient billing staff looked at me in disbelief, and I spent the entire day with them. The following Saturday I arrived and asked if someone would like to compete with me in the number of accounts billed. One young lady immediately volunteered, and we all worked in high gear the total day. I was trying to build my trust with them and deliberately billed fewer accounts than my competitor who looked victorious at the final count. I said, "So, I am second best. I was competing with a professional." I played this little game for a few weeks until we got caught up. I made some new friends in the process by getting into the trenches and working with them and injecting a little humor in the process. I viewed them as good folks, and the negativity disappeared with the backlog. It was one of the joys of just being part of the team and being a good player.

Sometime later, another hospital sent a couple of their representatives for a visit to our business office to overview our departments. When they arrived in the outpatient billing unit they asked about our billing backlog. Every one of my folks looked at me as I said, "We have no backlog!" The visitors were in shock and told us that they were always weeks behind. Upon their departure I did "thumbs up" to my outpatient billing group, and they chuckled with pride. Again, these are the joys of working with good people—teamwork!

My newly assigned billing supervisor could best be described complimentarily as a worker bee. As new employees were hired, they spent about six weeks sitting near her as she taught them the basics of billing. We had a large hemodialysis unit that required special billing procedures in which she was an expert. Many third-party payers would often refer the billing staff of other hemodialysis units to her for billing instruction. She was great. Also, she closely monitored any third-party payer mail-backs (identifying unpaid claims that required resubmission) to review with her staff to correct the billing to ensure prompt payment. Unfortunately, I learned that in many other hospitals the mail-backs were not given priority status and were subject to intermediary rejection.

In working with the supervisors under my direction, I tried to identify their strengths and weaknesses. My new billing supervisor believed that, if you billed correctly, the claim should be paid without further ado (mail-backs being the exception). It didn't work that way, and I took the necessary steps to see that appropriate follow-up of the unpaid accounts was timely. I usually worked at least sixty hours per week, which included weekends as well. I was very much involved in the day-to-day activities and had an open-door policy; I kept busy and "in tune." I allocated time every week to monitor billed and unbilled claims to ensure that they were being appropriately worked and not just sitting in limbo.

This process included identifying any slowness in payment by a specific insurance carrier or intermediary. Maintaining our accounts receivable at a favorable level was an ongoing priority to me. I was blessed with a wonderful assistant,

Erna, who performed those functions in unison with me. I had allocated certain sections of the billing unit for special considerations—one being unresolved claims resulting from third-party payer changes. Erna accepted special auditing assignments with alacrity and her thoroughness was evident.

When a new Medi-Cal intermediary took over, it was a nightmare getting old claims paid. Their lack of refinement seemed to drag in the submission of new claims. It was imperative that we follow closely with the intermediary, regardless of the ongoing "screw-ups" that were caused by the transition. Failure to perform ongoing timely follow-up procedures could cause claim rejections, regardless of the circumstances. Invariably, the intermediary habitually placed the onus on us.

I recall attending a Medi-Cal intermediary meeting in which they tried to tell us that they were current in processing our claims. These meetings are attended by billing personnel, and no one can "BS" them. There was an outcry at the meeting refuting their statement that their claims were current. Unfortunately for the speaker, he said, "I want someone here to provide a list of unpaid old claims not processed."

I stood up and walked to the podium with my package of unpaid claims and said, "Here they are!" The audience of billing personnel screamed with laughter and gave me a standing ovation. Again, don't mess with those folks—they know their business.

It became somewhat of a trend among key personnel who were employed by the intermediary to strike out on their own as specialized consultants. Being knowledgeable of the internal workings of their prior employer, they sought to represent the hospital in resolving unpaid claims. Because of the frustration in the resolution of these claims when new intermediaries entered the field, I felt vindictive enough to respond to those so-called specialists who were seeking to act on our behalf. I responded to one former staff member stating that, when employed by the intermediary, he did little to assist us in reconciling unpaid claims, and I felt he was quite audacious in offering his consulting services.

However, I believe that when proficient individuals become self-employed and offer their expertise relating to their former employer to others, their input can be very beneficial. I have used such persons pertaining to information systems for special projects. I found that those select individuals not only offer their general knowledge of their former employer's system, but also have worked with other hospitals that were faced with similar internal situations. By energizing their combined efforts, they can address and resolve issues and offer alternative solutions. Many of these folks come with storehouses of knowledge and can resolve difficult ongoing situations they previously encountered at other client sites.

I selected my credit supervisor Rose for her loyalty, tenacious work ethic, and total dedication to the department. She understood the necessity of ongoing follow-up procedures to maintain our accounts receivable at a satisfactory level. She was, however, a "diamond in the rough" and a handful at times. When she received her promotion she met with her staff. Their enthusiasm over her promotion was equivalent to enthusiasm for the Death March of Bataan during World War II.

After working with her for a while, however, the troops settled down, worked hard, and came to love and respect her. Her area of responsibility was private-pay accounts and those accounts with balances remaining after insurance, which were payable by the patient and/or other sources such as liens, estates, etc. Unresolved accounts were sent to the collection agency and we monitored their collection activity by performing unscheduled on-site random periodic audits. Unannounced, Rose and I simply arrived and took a list of accounts to review, and the collection agency never took umbrage. Rose and I worked on special projects together with good results.

One of the ladies who worked in the credit department was Janet. She was a Southern belle, married to a nice husband, and they had two sons. She was in her late thirties when I arrived at the hospital. In terms of appearance she was always trying to improve herself to be certain she reached her pinnacle—hair, makeup, dress, figure. To me, she was very feminine and always looked great. She had a very flirtatious nature and a sweet way about herself. We all loved her and teased her constantly in adoration. On one occasion, I was sitting with her at her desk helpfully giving her pointers in working her monthly follow-up of open accounts. In the process, she silently detected a touch of sternness in the tone of my voice. Her Southern background and manners rejected confrontation as she always put her best foot forward, so to speak. It was apparent to me she came from a very loving and caring family. That was confirmed when her sister and family came for a visit.

She jokingly said, "All the girls are jealous because you're sitting with me!"

I felt like Mark Twain's Tom Sawyer. She thought I was reprimanding her, and I said, "I am trying to be helpful because I love you so much."

She responded, "Forget the reprimand and just love me less."

My niece Robin and I went to Vancouver on vacation. A close friend and his company had just completed a magnificent high-rise at the harbor's edge and the royal couple, Charles and Diana, were coming to Vancouver for the opening, and also to attend the World's Fair. Robin and I were both excited about the trip. Before I left, Janet asked that I send her a postcard from Vancouver. I sent her a card as promised with the following message:

> The tulips are red and the grass is green,
> Vancouver in spring is a beautiful scene,
> While I may not be fluent in prose or pen,
> In the bow wow department, I think you're a ten.

Janet, being a good scout and knowing my silliness, got a kick out of her card and verse and all of her co-workers made copies. They all thought it was funny.

Much later, Janet had a facelift and requested of me another poem to celebrate the success of her surgery. (It seems I had unofficially become the poor man's Poet Laureate of SJRMC.) By the way, Janet's legal Christian name was Olene.

> Olene, Olene, you gorgeous queen,
> They say you're looking like a teen,
> They say the wrinkles have gone anew,
> You have even lost a chin or two,
> They say you're really looking swell,
> You always were a sexy gal.
> Life gets tough as time marches,
> All of those bags and fallen arches,
> When I say this, I don't mean maybe,
> You will always be, our bow wow baby.

She liked it and said, "I knew that last line would show up!" I love teasing people whom I truly adore and she certainly got more than her share. She was a great lady with a sunny disposition. She was loved by all and was always extremely attractive.

When I first started at SJRMC, two of my key employees were disenchanted with their supervisor, who had recently been hired to supervise two important departmental units. These two employees came to see me daily regarding this person and requesting resolution. They sensed that I was procrastinating in addressing the situation, which was becoming untenable and frustrating to them.

Being new, and apart from my own general orientation, it became apparent that I seriously needed to address their concerns. I carefully gathered and closely reviewed the information. I informed the CFO and the assistant CFO that I would have to discharge the supervisor in order to establish harmony within those units. In the process, I took all of the preliminary steps to justify the dismissal. I was very concerned and unhappy to perform this burdensome task. I was just getting my feet wet, figuratively speaking, and working with my staff and on numerous other pressing departmental issues.

I arranged a meeting with the supervisor at the end of the day and explained my unhappy mission. In the process, I went into great detail regarding this situation and her relationship with her employees.

The meeting was not contentious but rather conciliatory, affording me the opportunity to candidly discuss her demeanor in depth. Never once during our discussion did she take umbrage by my comments and observations. When we finished our meeting, her husband was to pick her up after work. She was without a car. As he did not arrive after our meeting, I volunteered to drive her home. It was a sadly quiet and awkward ride for both of us.

I had prearranged that, after the meeting, I would meet the assistant CFO at the driving range at one of our local golf courses. When I arrived late, I explained the situation to him and I was glad that he had waited to hit some balls. I was quite upset and unhappy to have had to perform such a miserable undertaking. He realized my concerns and was supportive by joining me at the driving range to spend some quiet time thereafter. It is beneficial to have someone you trust to commiserate with after performing such an ordeal.

Three brothers were physicians at SJRMC, and each had his own established practice. They had a cousin, Dr. Jay, who was currently the medical director of a rehabilitation unit at Baylor University Hospital in Texas. His cousins at SJRMC coaxed him to move to California and to come to our hospital. Upon his arrival, he met with our CFO who asked me to also attend their meeting. After meeting Dr. Jay, the CFO suggested that I help him get established and do whatever it took—in very broad terms. Fortunately, I immediately liked the doctor and I was happy to work with him.

I arranged a billing service for him to get the ball rolling in establishing his individual provider numbers with all leading third-party payers. Additionally, I took him to all of the key intermediaries, starting with Blue Cross of California, who, aside from their plans, administered the Medicare program as well as several others. Those visits mainly focused on patient care, reporting, and protocol—all very important topics to ensure the processing of our claims and timely reimbursement. Additionally, I had him meet with the Ventura County Medi-Cal administrative team to cover their protocol. The overall intention was to establish a working relationship and determine that, in terms of treatment and protocol, everyone was on the same page.

I quickly learned that working with Dr. Jay was no difficult task. He presented himself affably when meeting others and was very frank when addressing the most basic bread-and-butter issues. From my observation during our visits, his treatment plan and protocol were widely and favorably received. We became very good colleagues and each of us viewed the other as someone who had his ducks in order as we diligently worked on our projects.

From my standpoint, it was very important to arrange meetings and luncheons with Workers' Compensation groups to let them know that Dr. Jay was starting a new unit at SJRMC and we would be eager to provide services to their patients. All of these activities were in the preliminary stages and I was eager to outline and plan the marketing stages of the program.

Meanwhile, an assistant administrator, John, had been assigned to oversee the establishment of the actual inpatient rehabilitation unit in conjunction with an outpatient services unit. John and I were to work closely together in getting our individual projects moving conjunctively. However, unlike Dr. Jay, John appeared rather remote in working with me. I sensed aloofness in his demeanor. It was obvious to me that John was proficient in executing his administrative duties. He had started his career as a pharmacist and he was in his mid-thirties. Occasionally my enthusiasm is misunderstood and that misjudgment has depicted me as being 95 percent conversation and 5 percent performance. (Although I am unable to attest to it personally, I had heard the same analogy applied to high-class hookers.)

After we got working together, John reversed those figures and we became good friends. As we progressed toward opening day for both units, John was extremely complimentary in recognizing my ongoing contribution to the hospital and, particularly, his units.

I, in keeping with the promotional plan, arranged a special luncheon for Workers' Compensation carriers at our hospital. I was promoting Dr. Jay's new department, along with another outpatient services department, whose director was Jane H. Both key persons were to speak and explain their services followed by a question-and-answer period. I expected and received a wonderful turnout of about one hundred persons. Prior to the meeting, my admitting manager Martha breezed into my office. She saw me writing notes on a pad. "Gus, are you writing notes for the meeting tomorrow?"

"Yes, Martha."

"Forget it. You are far more effective when you just speak off the cuff."

"Do you really think so?"

"I know so. Just get up there and do your thing and forget all of this paper stuff."

"Thanks!"

The following day, the luncheon was well attended, as predicted. I apparently made a good presentation on all of the services that we were attempting to promote. However, in introducing our first guest speaker, I ran into a somewhat very embarrassing problem. "Ladies and Gentleman, I am pleased to introduce Jane … Jane?"

Quick thinking and considerate, Jane stood and said, "You know, Gus, you remind me of my husband, Tarzan. He forever says, 'Me Tarzan, you Jane.'" The audience gave Jane a thunderous round of applause, complete with laughter. She saved my hide and turned my stumble into a hilarious event.

The meeting was a success and I learned my lesson: always write down the names.

After the luncheon, I stopped by the CFO's office to critique the meeting. A senior vice president (another Jane, by the way) was already in his office discussing the meeting. When an opening occurred in their conversation, I quickly, asked the following:

"Jane, did you tell Don about my faux pas forgetting Jane's surname?"

"No, Gus. I told him that you stood in front of the podium and delivered the most dynamic speech without a single note. No one stands before an audience of over one hundred persons and delivers a speech such as yours, just off the cuff. I was just telling Don how amazing you are in capturing your audience so effectively."

"Jane, thanks for your kind words. Martha told me to just get up there and talk. But never again will I go before an audience without having written down the names of the speakers following me. I learned my lesson—I felt so stupid. Luckily, Tarzan's Jane bailed me out this time."

We all worked hard to get our rehab unit off the ground. I had Dr. Jay work with my admitting and patient representatives, educating them on all pre-admission requirements and other information regarding obtaining authorizations and so forth. The inpatient unit immediately started running with a very high census and the outpatient unit did as well. We worked in concert and really achieved our goals in getting Dr. Jay on board and establishing our inpatient and outpatient rehabilitation services.

John was the assistant administrator who was assigned to work with me on the Dr. Jay project. He was a tennis player and his wife was a registered nurse in our intensive care unit. They had tennis courts in their condominium and John's wife was an excellent gourmet cook and wonderful pastry chef. What a great combination—good friends and tennis followed by a delicious dinner. My visits with them were very enjoyable. John's wife always sent me home with a bag of scrumptious fresh pastries. My relationship with John had had a precarious start, but he turned out to be one of my greatest fans—filling me with lavish praise at every opportunity. I praised him in kind.

A few weeks after we got the units in operation, Dr. Jay and I called upon the medical director of a rehab unit in the San Fernando Valley. We were hoping to make a reciprocal arrangement with the medical director on joint referrals. After our introductions, the doctor was very cordial but extremely forthright in expressing his thoughts. "Dr. Jay, what the hell are you doing with this guy—he is in the enemy camp!"

"No, Gus is my best friend."

Dr. Jay turned to me and we both laughed; we thought it was pretty funny.

However, the other doctor's point may have been well taken, as persons in my position can be considered—fairly or unfairly—stumbling blocks.

15

An important goal for me at SJRMC was to stabilize our staffing complement, as I addressed earlier. I personally hired several new persons and everything seemed to settle down. One lady, whom I had initially hired, developed the problem of having the inability to concentrate on her work. I arranged for her and her supervisor to meet with me.

"Cheryl, I have noticed that you seem to have a problem maintaining focus in performing your billing duties."

"Mr. Munro, I don't understand what you are talking about."

"You seem to be fidgeting all of the time. You seem to be looking about, moving about, and not concentrating on your work for longer than three or four minutes, and off you go again."

"I have no idea what you are talking about and I feel rather offended by your observation and your accusations."

"Cheryl, you have clearly emphasized your thoughts in my direction. However, having worked with me for some time, would it seem logical to you that I would simply call you into my office this afternoon, just to criticize you?"

"No, you wouldn't!"

"I want to help you. I would like you to move your work to the vacant desk, outside my office across from my secretary."

"Oh, the hot seat."

Me, laughingly, "Oh, is that what they call it?"

Cheryl, also laughingly, "Oh dear, what will the gang think seeing me in the hot seat."

"Tell them it is a signal of endearment, between you and me."

"Oh, yes, right!"

Later the following day, Cheryl stopped me as I entered my office, "Mr. Munro, I want to talk with you for a couple of minutes."

"Come on in now."

"I was really annoyed at you during our meeting. But I realize that you have treated us all so fairly. I just couldn't identify your observations until this morning. I sat down, and in a few minutes I started to fidget again—exactly what you said. I am working on it and I am going to stop this bad pattern."

Shortly thereafter, during the holiday season, some former patients were stopping by my office with gifts galore. We had a practice of not accepting gifts; however, I made exceptions as these persons were so grateful and wanted to express their appreciation. I especially took into account those persons who were presenting me with handmade items—it would be offensive for me to refuse these.

One lady brought me one of her handmade couch throws, and it was really nice. Being in the infamous hot seat, Cheryl could clearly see what was going on with my deluge of gifts. When these types of situations occur, it has always behooved me to discuss unusual incidents, selectively, with members of my staff. I motioned her to come into my office.

"Mr. Munro, look at all of the beautiful gifts you have been receiving. I am impressed."

"Frankly, I try to discourage them. Technically, I shouldn't be receiving them. Look at this beautiful throw. She would be offended if I didn't accept it!"

"I agree, and it is so beautiful."

"You probably think that I have been hoodwinking these folks as you know the real me—a real SOB."

"Mr. Munro, don't say that. You're not."

"Cheryl, you are back on track and doing great. I am proud of you. Do you want to move out of the infamous hot seat?"

"No, I am staying here and keeping you out of trouble—all of those ladies bringing you gifts."

"Are you serious about remaining in the hot seat?"

"Absolutely!"

"You are a sweetheart, and I love you."

"Mr. Munro, I love you too."

The hospital temporarily hired a CFO to work with our administrative team on certain projects to accommodate him until he found a permanent position elsewhere. It seemed to me that he must have been highly thought of to receive this consideration.

One day he had some free time and decided to come to my office and rattle my cage. He sat down and asked me about our billing and follow-up system and exactly what steps I took to monitor assurance that the accounts receivable were being managed in a timely and effective manner. This meeting took place prior to the advanced computerization of accounts receivable.

He looked at shelving outside of my office in the credit department unit and asked if they housed the open accounts. I responded affirmatively, and he asked that I randomly select about fifteen accounts for him to review. He could see me clearly pulling the accounts randomly, and I simply handed them to him. He reviewed each one and said, "What are CR1, CR2, etc.?" Additionally, he reviewed the notes on the accounts, made note of patients making partial monthly payments, and pulled copies of letters in the individual patient jacket.

I explained our CR letter series, stamp, and comments.

When he finished, he stood up and shook my hand and said, "Wow, I am impressed."

I mentioned his visit to the CFO, who said, "What the hell is he doing looking in your department?"

I quoted that old expression, "One look is worth a thousand words."

The hospital wanted to add a financial specialist to our board of directors. The candidate they chose held an executive position with a company commercially quite unrelated to the healthcare industry and our hospital. As soon as he became a board member, he seemed to become very vocal regarding the status of our accounts receivable. He strongly believed that all of our open accounts should be paid within less than thirty days—without exception. (This was prior to online billing.) As part of the collection process, we had to furnish copies of our operative reports and discharge summaries to certain insurance carriers and we were dependent on physician dictation and medical records transcription procedures. I kept hearing his comments each month criticizing the status of our accounts receivable.

After about three months, I suggested that he come to see me to review my department. He came and I pulled the individual accounts and explained our billing and follow-up procedures step by step. I explained that we had pending categories with large balances—such as patients who had applied for Medi-Cal and were awaiting approval. It took up to ninety days or longer to obtain approval. As a reputable businessman in the community, he was entitled to a better understanding of the issues and ramifications of billing practices and third-party processing procedures. I welcomed the opportunity to discuss the topic in length, which was a wasted effort as he was looking for a quick fix without the boring details.

Shortly after arriving at SJRMC, I met a young lady who was working in our emergency room in both the reception unit and in the physicians' back office. Those persons in the registration unit in that department reported to me. I immediately thought she sort of resembled my ex-wife. Some of her positive mannerisms sort of reminded me slightly of her. Unlike my ex-wife, she appeared to me to be slightly standoffish toward me when we first met. I realized, in all fairness to her, that my assessment may have been too premature.

She was divorced and eleven years younger than I. She was the mother of two young daughters and, apparently, was seriously dating one of our physicians, a married man. I had started at the hospital in February and at coffee break with the assistant CFO, I informed him that I would be marrying this young lady before the end of the year.

We were married in December in Carmel. The day we returned home, her jilted physician called to state that he and his wife were getting a divorce. She had to tell him she had just returned from her honeymoon.

The following week, while standing in the cafeteria line, my good friend (?) the assistant CFO, saw the former boyfriend standing in front of me and he patted his shoulder and fled away. The jilted lover turned and saw me. Awkwardly I managed to mutter, "Hi, how are you?" It was so embarrassing—but funny—and I could have kicked the little bugger, the assistant CFO, for pulling that prank. Talk about perfect timing!

I always realized that the medical records department was a most important contributor to the success of patient accounts for many reasons. I particularly had a kinship for persons performing the medical record transcriptions.

Needless to say, they required a commanding vocabulary and the ability to decipher what the physician is conveying—particularly when English may be a second language. The kinship correlation refers to my days as a communications operator and supervisor at the Canadian Pacific Railway. My only medical challenge at the Canadian Pacific Railway had been to correctly spell the "ABC Pharmaceutical Company," which was a handful for this grade-school dropout.

In our medical records department we had a wonderful gifted lady who had an exemplary talent for performing transcription functions. However—in plain English—she was as nutty as a fruitcake. With all of her talent, she was not playing with a full deck so to speak. She was aggressive, obstreperous, and foulmouthed. She could tell you to go to hell without batting an eye. For some strange reason, she thought I was great, and I hoped that the old adage "opposites attract" could be considered valid. When she received any medical bills or similar paperwork from the hospital or a physician's office, she would stop by my office, waiving any of the amenities, such as checking with my assistant or secretary before seeing me, and just simply barge in unannounced.

"Mr. Munro, look at this goddamn bill. What the hell is going on?"

I would patiently but forcefully respond, "Helen, look at me and please listen. I will take care of this situation. Don't worry about it. If you receive any more bills, simply give them to my secretary or leave them on my desk should I be out of the office."

When seeing me throughout the complex and in the company of others, she would point to me and say to them proudly, "That man runs this whole place. And he and I are very good friends."

My wife, as the coordinator in the emergency services department, worked closely with the medical staff and admitting representatives. At that time, the medical director of that department had his wife performing certain administrative tasks on his behalf. The doctor's wife, was a great person, very intelligent and definitely very hip! She had a great sense of humor and was down to earth. One morning she walked into my wife's unit and said, "Some old dame met me on the stairway and informed me that I was nothing but a goddamn slut!"

My wife screamed and said, "You have just informally met Helen."

When my wife conveyed this tale to me, my cheeks were sore for a day from laughing.

Before I met my second wife, and during my initial orientation at the hospital, I met with one of the directors who had substantial responsibilities. At the close of our meeting, she asked if I would like to accompany her to a forthcoming hospital event. I sort of left her invitation hanging, politely explaining, "I'll get back to you later."

After leaving her office, I stopped by to see the assistant CFO with a question: "Hi, I just met with Beth and wondered, what is her story?"

"She has a lot of responsibility and performs well."

"At the end of our meeting, she asked me for a date."

"What! She dates the director, Hector. He goes to her house after work and on the weekends and fixes up her home. I can't believe what you are saying."

"She wants me to accompany her to the awards dinner."

"That poor guy is working his ass off on her house. This is unbelievable."

"Don't worry, I'll bow out. Thank God I spoke with you. This could have been embarrassing to all."

"So you are turning out to be Mr. Prince Charming! Ha, Ha!"

"Shut up, you little brat." Before leaving, we looked at each other and laughed, as he was shaking his head in disbelief over this conversation.

One day much later, I was speaking with Beth in the hallway and we were standing in front of my wife's office. Her door was open and she saw us in conversation. I heard an overhead page for me and I excused myself from Beth and returned to my office. I called the operator in response to the page and she said to call my wife.

"Did you just call me?"

"Yes!"

"Why? I was standing right in front of your door talking with Beth."

"That woman is after you and I couldn't just sit there and do nothing."

"Jealous?"

"Yes!"

I thought it was pretty funny and it put me in a playful mood. Later, I went to my wife's office. "What are you doing for lunch, young lady?"

"Nothing special."

I winked at her and said, "Let's go home, skip the lunch, and just have dessert."

She laughingly said, "Call me when you're ready to leave."

"You are serious about this proposal, aren't you?"

"Yes, indeed!"

"You just get back to business and we'll postpone this proposal until after work."

Said she with a wink, "Better late than never!"

Unfortunately, and very sadly, it was all too short a relationship. I did not relate to her children and it simply did not work out. Meanwhile, the jilted doctor married an attractive radiologist thereafter and he and I developed a nice rapport.

I received an important letter from one of my healthcare colleagues, who was very actively involved in all activities relating to third-party payers. He himself served a group of hospitals and I thought very highly of him. He stated that one of our major insurance carriers was about to limit our interim billing for patients who remain in the hospital for longer periods of time.

Ongoing interim billing was an important procedure for prolonged stays to keep our cash flow routinely flowing. As this was a major issue, a special meeting was planned, to be followed by a meeting with the major insurance provider. We were encouraged to attend both meetings and forward our comments in advance. I fired off a letter explaining the need to retain this procedure and bulleted the salient points. Because it was an important issue, I decided to meet with the hospital group and attend their meeting and then meet with the intermediary thereafter.

I was surprised to learn, as we started our preliminary meeting, that my letter was distributed to all of the attendees as the basis of their presentation. That being the case, I suggested that I be actively involved in making the presentation. I did attend important meetings that usually included various speakers from within the healthcare industry, including my management team. As this meeting had been prepared in advance, I was surprised, as a last-minute participant, that the presentation was solely based on my documentation. What pleased me most was that I was totally in tune to these situations and my criteria had been based on my own observations. We met with the provider and some concessions were made.

At the end of each month, before our month-end financial cutoff, I attempted to apply every single payment I could get my hands on to help reduce our days in accounts receivable. It was a general formula measurement of comparing one hospital to another, and every payment helped to reduce our days outstanding.

If we experienced a particularly slow cash payment month, I would make a concerted effort to obtain additional payments before the cutoff. I would contact third-party payers to expedite additional payments, make certain all of our mail containing payments had been picked up from the post office, etc. Whatever I was able to gather, I would run it through our cash processing in data processing and they, in turn, would put it through the system before the month ended.

I had been working with a patient regarding her insurance off and on for a couple of months. The lady had an ongoing illness and she was very concerned regarding her insurance and other medical issues. She was extremely reserved and businesslike, but I could tell that she respected my opinion. I surmised that she was grateful for my assistance and intervention in helping her. All of my meetings with her had been conducted while she was hospitalized, and I would visit her in her hospital room.

One day, I was rushing to take the month-end payments to the cashier's office. I hurried to the main hospital entrance and, as I went to enter the door, I heard a woman's voice calling me. I turned and saw this lady, who was accompanied by her daughter. I looked and paused for a moment, and without thinking said, "Oh hello, Mrs. S, I'm sorry I just didn't recognize you with your clothes on."

"Mr. Munro!" Mrs. S. exclaimed.

Her daughter, who had never met me, went hysterical over my stupid comment.

Feeling myself blush, I moved quickly into the building. I was so embarrassed as I rushed to get the payments processed. Fortunately, her daughter's laughter helped save the day.

The lady had come to be readmitted to the hospital. I sheepishly stopped by her room the following day and said, "Mrs. S your daughter must think you are associating with some really unsavory individuals, me in particular."

Mrs. S responded, "Mr. Munro, my daughter thinks you are so funny." With her comments came a half-smile that was very generous for a very reserved lady. It meant I was off the hook.

I unexpectedly received a belated compliment regarding my tenure at The Hospital of the Good Samaritan. I had the occasion to visit the district credit manager, whom I had known at Richfield. The company was now ARCO and he was located in their twin towers, former site of the old Richfield gold dome building. This was a sad pilgrimage, seeing this ultra-modern structure which had replaced our beautiful art deco building that had been so dominating in the old Los Angeles skyline.

He was currently under medical care with one of the physicians at Good Samaritan. He said that he casually mentioned my name to his doctor to see if he had known me while I was employed at Good Samaritan.

The credit manager, said, "Gus, the doctor spoke of you throughout my total visit to his office by stating that you had made a great contribution to the hospital, patients, and physicians and their office personnel. It was almost like you walked on water, he was so impressed with you!"

His comments pleased me very much. He and I had worked closely together at Richfield. A number of the management team had been very upset at my decision to leave that corporation. My friend's physician at Good Samaritan had always been so supportive of me and sort of in the vanguard of my fan club. He always freely expressed positive comments regarding my work in general and my work with patients in particular to the administrative staff and board members. He was an excellent physician in the field of pulmonary medicine.

St. John's has a very large hemodialysis unit. Because of the substantial amount of services involved and the financial implications, I worked very closely with this unit. One of my favorite patients was a Mr. R, who was a soft-spoken and very kind black gentleman. He quite frequently used a wheel chair and he had a young man assisting his needs most of the time. Late one afternoon, I ran into them in the hall en route to admitting. They had just come from the doctor's office and Mr. R. needed to be admitted. I accompanied them to admitting and checked to see if we had received a request to admit from the doctor's office.

We had received no admitting orders, and, as the patient was physically in discomfort, I took him directly to the nursing unit where he would normally be admitted. The nurse on duty said they had no admitting orders and she proceeded to call the doctor. As the patient was safe in the unit, I simply returned to my office, but wondered why we had received no orders in advance of the patient.

The following morning, as I was walking down the hall, I saw two doctors hysterically laughing. Excitedly, they stopped me. One said, "Gus, we just heard the good news! You have been granted admitting privileges."

The other one exclaimed, "Gus you are the only non-physician on staff with those privileges. Outstanding!"

Totally bewildered but laughingly I said, "Honestly, I don't know what you are talking about." I walked on leaving them still laughing. I could think of nothing in correlation with their comments.

We all worked hard, but we had a lot fun at the hospital. I ignored their comments. I thought they were putting me on. About half an hour later, I received a call from Mr. R's doctor, who informed me that I did a wonderful job for the hospital, but that I had to stop admitting his patients. I learned that the patient had had an appointment with his physician and, after leaving his office to go home, he became ill. Instead of returning to the doctor's office and seeking medical assistance and resolution, he circumvented the procedure and came directly to the hospital. When greeting Mr. R, I was totally unaware of the facts.

Upon receiving Mr. R's physician's call, I suddenly realized why those two physicians had been laughing so hysterically. Needless to say, it was a close-knit place.

However, my solace and vindication was that I got the admitting diagnosis correctly. Out of necessity, he was hospitalized for five days. Regardless, my admitting privileges couldn't be revoked, as they were non-existent anyway. Ha!

One day I ran into Mr. R in the hallway as he was en route to the hemodialysis unit. He spoke to me and said that his vision was very poor and that he had difficulty seeing. Trying to be encouraging I said, "Well, you saw me."

He laughed and said, "You walk so quickly down the halls—almost running—that I recognized you by movement." I received those comments all of the time about running down the halls.

As he was a diabetic, the condition of his poor sight was apparently not uncommon. I prayed for the restoration of his sight each day. Sometime later, one of the nuns who worked in the hemodialysis unit stopped by my office to give me some updates on some of our patients. During our conversation, I asked Sister, "How is my good friend, Mr. R progressing?"

She replied, "Gus, a strange thing has happened. His sight is slowly being restored."

I didn't want a Sister of Mercy to know that I had been messing in their business, but I do believe in the power of prayer.

Well, now that I have gotten started, I may as well continue on my nun stories. One Saturday I was working and I decided to stir up the pot. I went to the gift shop and selected a valentine. I addressed it to our sister administrator and signed the CFO's name.

I involved one of the assistant administrators, also a sister, in the plot. She accepted the valentine and placed it on the sister's breakfast table the following morning, Sunday, Valentine's Day.

Monday morning, the CFO came running into my office asking if I knew anything about a valentine. I played dumb, which comes easy. He handed me a Peanuts cartoon, sent to him by the sister administrator (valentine recipient) in which Lucy is asking the question, "Do you send valentines to people you hate?"

The sister added a note of thanks to the CFO for the valentine. The CFO, being a good sport (?), said to me, "I will fire whoever sent that valentine and your name is prominently on my suspect list."

Disregarding his comment, I grabbed the Peanuts cartoon and made copies and handed it back to him saying, "This is so funny."

Innocently pretending to get onboard the bandwagon, I thoughtfully suggested to him, "It was probably your administrative golf buddy who sent it."

The golf buddy arrived in my office shortly after the CFO's departure and said, "You SOB, you sent that G-D valentine. Do you realize the CFO doesn't even send his wife one?"

I said, "There is a message there."

We let him stew for a couple of days and the sister administrator stopped by my office. With a twinkle in her eye and said, "Gus, we have to tell the CFO the truth."

I said, "Sister, I will, with the proviso that you enter his office first and leave last."

After my confession, the CFO said, "Gus, it appeared to be one of your pranks, but I just wasn't certain. Had I known it was you I would have reciprocated with one of mine."

For several years the CFO and I sent sister a valentine each year. The year she became the mother general at Burlingame we sent her a collect telegram valentine. She never lost her sense of humor and always reciprocated every Valentine's Day. Aside from being extremely dynamic in her role as a sister, she was, incredibly, a very beautiful lady with a kind heart and a tremendous sense of humor. She was very businesslike and a perfectionist and you earned your close relationship with her by performing your duties by exemplifying her high standards.

Shortly after the valentine incident, the director of plant and equipment, who could best be described as a "Nosy Parker" (busybody), sent a memorandum to key departments regarding the main floor men's restroom.

In the memorandum he stated that the urinal was unpredictable and did not always function properly. He suggested that, temporarily, as my office was across the hall from the restroom, I should check periodically to be certain all was well. Prior to his memorandum I knew nothing of his intent regarding his proposed solution. I made a copy of his memorandum and sent it to Sister, commenting facetiously that if that assignment was listed on my job description, it must have been written in the small print. Sister was delighted with this situation and immediately responded in her humorous fashion. The administrative golf buddy immediately got on the bandwagon and had a standard desk name plate made that said: A. R. Munro, VP of Latrines. He brought the administrative team to my office to make the formal presentation. After the valentine prank, it was get-even time.

Sister had arranged a special management meeting at a banquet restaurant for an all-day workshop and luncheon. I attended with my then wife, who was also a member of the management team. I excused myself during a break in the program to go to the restroom. With such a large crowd attending, unmarked auxiliary restrooms were made available across from the main building. I went into one of the facilities to find the cubical being used. I waited in the standing area near the wash basin for the occupant to leave the cubical. I had assumed it was another man, but when sister opened the door and our faces met, I suffered from total embarrassment and astonishment. "Excuse me," said I, while running out so she could use the wash basin.

I awkwardly decided to wait until she came by. I had never been confronted with a situation such as this one before. I was totally unprepared to determine the best course of action to take—if any. At those shocking moments, I was devoid of any sense of humor.

Smilingly and nonchalantly she breezed by saying, "No problem, Gus, it is coed!"

When I returned to my wife, she said somewhat impatiently, "What kept you?"

"I just went to the restroom with Sister." I had to sit with my wife the rest of the day as she was shaking with glee.

When I told the CFO, he said "You will be a major dinner topic at the nunnery tonight."

Previously, my wife had mentioned that she had the occasion to drive with sister to a meeting in Ventura. She said Sister drove like a maniac, and that her heart had been in her mouth the whole trip. I remembered her comments when, one Saturday morning at work, Sister dropped by and said, "I heard that you purchased a new automobile."

"Yes!"

"Gus, let's go look at it now."

When I showed her the car, she said, "Gus I love it. It's an automatic—may I take us for a spin in and around our campus?" What could I say?

When we finished she looked at me and said, "Were you frightened of my driving?"

I said, "Oh no!"

Said she, "Why did you have your hands on the door, just ready to jump?" I decided to remain speechless.

Late one afternoon, I stopped by her office to see if she was available for a short humorous chat. Jokingly I said, "I hope you realize all of the good things I do for this hospital and the Sisters of Mercy."

"I do, and you know that, Gus!"

"Well, I have just been asked to go on a date with widow X, our key volunteer who runs the gift shop. She is over seventy and I am but forty-four years old!"

Sister replied, "WHAT!" We both started to laugh and I asked facetiously that she revise my job description to exclude certain social events.

I did mention that a lot of the older influential families, who had had ties to our hospital and supported our mission, should be there. Sister said, "What are you going to do?"

I replied, "I am going on that date and I will be thinking of you laughing at me and telling the other sisters of my dilemma."

"Gus, that is nice of you to escort her." She, laughed, but I knew she approved.

And, one more Nun story. One of my favorite, and somewhat mischievous, persons in the order stopped by my office to see if I wanted anything from the local library. We had a lot of fun together and I asked her what she was reading and returning to the library. She had five books and handed them to me. There were a couple on religion and a couple on general topics. The fifth one, however, was *How to Burglarize a Home.*

"What is this?" I said.

She laughed and said that it was so fascinating learning the tricks of the trade, she could hardly put the book down at bedtime. I believe the author of that book was a former thief who had gone straight. She was a scream, and this is but one example.

16

For me, working with personnel in physicians' offices was always paramount in developing and maintaining good working relationships within the hospital. As in any other business, their staffing complement periodically changes. It was important for me to keep up with those changes, always knowing whom to call and work with closely. To begin with, I was a little slow in developing luncheons and group meetings with the physicians' office personnel. During that period, within our hospital as well as within our industry, achieving goals by specific yearly objectives became very popular and the norm.

I decided to submit a commitment to maintain closer working relationships with our physicians' office personnel in my formalized yearly objectives. Shortly after joining the hospital, I did have a luncheon for them, and it was very productive. Unfortunately, my commitment to having these luncheons periodically was short lived due to ongoing pressing projects and issues.

To fulfill my formalized commitment, I arranged for a physicians' luncheon and developed an interesting program of topics to be discussed. It was a wonderful turnout of about ninety-five persons, an overwhelming response. When starting the meeting, I viewed it importantly and, with slight embarrassment, mentioned that, at our last meeting, we unanimously had agreed that it would be appropriate to meet regularly. I sheepishly put my arm at my face level and said, "That was months and months ago." Thankfully, they roared at my comments and gestures. Fortunately, it was a very successful and productive meeting.

A few weeks later, a manager of one of the larger medical offices called me. "Hi, Gus. Are you ready for a bizarre conversation?"

"Why not!"

"Gus, we have a select group of ladies, all from our medical offices, and we on, a regular basis, meet socially."

"That's great!"

"At our last dinner, we asked one of the ladies, who is soon to celebrate her birthday, what she would like for a gift. The lady responded, 'A date with Gus Munro!' We all laughed and said we would see if it could be arranged."

"Wow, who is the lady?"

"Her name is Judy [I'm giving her a fictitious name here] and she works for Doctor X. You may not recall her, but she did attend the recent luncheon."

"I would probably recognize her if I saw her."

"She is very attractive, separated from her husband, and very interested in you. She is impressed with your looks and appearance and says your shoes are well shined."

"That is very complimentary. I don't recall her, but I have heard about the shoes before."

"Gus, are you interested in taking her on a date?"

"Why not!"

"We have pooled our money and the evening is on us. Thanks for being a good sport. We'll get back to you with the details."

"Sounds great!"

We met and I remembered having seen her at the luncheon. She was very attractive, well groomed, had excellent manners and good conversation skills. However, it was doomed from the start.

She asked if I knew her ex who operated a shuttle service for our patients with infirmities. I was shocked to learn that I knew him based on mutual patient issues regarding his services. He was very affable and provided good services to our patients and the community. It kind of put a damper on the evening and I thought it would be dreadful should we happen to run into him. Oxnard was a small place.

Regardless of the circumstances, I could not accept a gratis evening and simply run off.

I called this lady a week or so later and suggested we have dinner in Woodland Hills and stop by and see my sister and family. She loved the idea and she enjoyed meeting my family, followed by the dinner thereafter. We somehow hopefully, sagaciously, and discreetly ended this brief acquaintanceship, although we met at meetings. I had a couple of visits to see her physician employer, as a patient. We always greeted each other warmly, and it had been a brief and interesting experience. I continued to work with her ex and had no feelings of guilt or remorse, and he apparently knew nothing of our brief encounter. I frankly was hopeful that they would reunite, as I liked them both very much.

One weekend, I had to attend four weddings—one on Friday evening and three on Saturday. They were all hospital employee related. The final one was between a part-time employee and her young man, who was learning to be a pilot as an avocation.

One year later, to celebrate their first wedding anniversary, the young pilot couple, along with their best man and maid of honor, flew a private plane to the San Fernando Valley for dinner. On the return flight, the best man requested to sit with the bridegroom pilot and the two ladies sat behind them. As they were descending to prepare to land at the Oxnard Airport, the plane suddenly hit some electrical wires and crashed. Both young men were killed instantly and both ladies very badly burned and immediately rushed to the burn center in Sherman Oaks.

On the following morning, which was Saturday, I was at the office when one of my employees gave me the shattering news. That afternoon I decided to drive to the burn unit.

I met the parents and family members of both young ladies. They were really pleased that I had arrived. The parents of my young employee Denise requested that I see her; she had just learned that her husband had been killed. Needless to say, this was a very sad and traumatic visit. I had felt somewhat hesitant in going to the hospital, but I wanted to pay my respects to all.

When I spoke with Denise, she asked that I keep her job open for her. I assured her not to worry about anything work-related, as we were all there to support her. I personally took over her work assignment, so that there would be no need to hire someone temporarily. I wanted her to be free to come back whenever she wanted to return. She required several months of skin grafting and she recovered physically very nicely. We learned that, at the time of the accident, she was about four-months pregnant and, fortunately, she was able to deliver a very healthy "miracle baby."

Several months passed, and she had received a sizeable settlement due to the accident; therefore, she decided to establish new goals and not to return to the hospital. She and her baby daughter came to see us to celebrate her recovery. We had a special luncheon for her. During lunch, while discussing her medical care, she stated that the skin grafts on her hands actually came from her backside. She said, "In other words, if some young man kisses my hand he is actually kissing my you-know-what." With all of her difficulties—loaded with pain, suffering and loss—it was a joy to share her humor.

It is my understanding that her friend made a good recovery as well. It was such a tragic situation for those two young ladies—losing their young men and having months of physical and emotional pain and ongoing treatment. We were amazed at how well our young lady recovered and gave birth to her beautiful little daughter.

Denise's work assignment primarily had been gathering reports and obtaining diagnoses from medical records for billing purposes. During the months that I assumed that responsibility, I learned, through osmosis, a tremendous amount about medical records. That department was an important element to the success of patient accounts. Also, the task enabled me to implement some beneficial procedural changes and options relating to the business office and medical records unit.

One morning, I received a telephone call from the former admitting and patient representative supervisor, whom I had had to dismiss shortly after my arrival at SJRMC. She sounded exceedingly effervescent and gracious in informing me who she was and that this telephone call was extremely important to her. Before commencing further she asked me if the timing was right. I responded, "Yes!"

Further, she inquired if I recalled the details of our conversation when we met that last day. I said, "Yes, vividly."

She warmly and fluently proceeded by stating, "I am so grateful to you for what you said to me at our last meeting. Your words were so profoundly expressed and instrumental in providing the impetus for me to finally seek help and to enroll in a twelve-step program." She spoke so kindly and appreciatively, it was a very riveting and gratifying experience for me to suddenly and very unexpectedly receive. I felt almost spellbound as her thoughts poured out so ebulliently.

She continued and exclaimed, "Throughout the program your words to me were so vivid and apropos—it was a reinforcing factor in my rehabilitation."

She went on to say that she and her husband had divorced. Further, she had met a wonderful man, also in the program. They were now happily married and living very productive lives. This was, unequivocally, one of the nicest messages that I had ever received. I cherish that call. We thereafter reunited socially.

Our sister administrator left SJRMC, being reassigned to fulfill another administrative position in San Francisco. Sister's position as administrator at SJRMC had been promotionally assigned to our vice president, Richard. He was a CPA and had a master's degree in hospital administration. He became the first lay administrator at SJRMC. He had worked closely with our sister administrator and the transition ran smoothly. Additionally, he had been actively involved in all departments and he was respected by all. Like Sister, he was totally committed to the hospital and the Mission of the Sisters of Mercy. It was a very happy place to work and continuity of administration was reassuring to both management and staff at SJRMC. He was in his mid-thirties and respected for his good business acumen and humanistic qualities.

The hospital acquired property that was adjacent to the hospital—across a back road behind our complex. It had formerly been a primary grade school. Acquiring this property, and particularly having the use of the buildings for storage, was really beneficial. I was very fortunate to be allocated one entire classroom to store our previous years' paid patient accounts in compliance with standard retention guidelines.

My credit supervisor Rose was extremely meticulous in overseeing our file management program. Along with her, we had been blessed with having a retired gentleman with a banking background who worked part-time to maintain our ongoing daily filing of paid accounts for the current fiscal year. We quickly transferred prior paid accounts to our new location, keeping the current year in the hospital's storage room. The retiree would periodically perform a cursory review from A to Z to verify correct filing. His work assignment was several rungs down his career ladder, but, being a team player, he accepted it with alacrity.

At the end of the year, Rose and two of her male part-time employees, who were students, and I would box the paid accounts and transfer them to the storeroom. Simultaneously, we would destroy the oldest prior year. As it was an arduous task I would wear casual clothes—tennis gear—when I helped work the transfer.

One day, Richard saw me and commented that my services were a little high priced for the manual transfer of accounts to storage. I was slightly taken back by his comment. It was really important to me to maintain good storage management. It was important, especially when immediate retrieval was required.

However, several months later, Richard and his administrative team did a walk-through on all of the storage classrooms. He was not happy making the rounds. Our file room was the only one in proper businesslike order. I was belatedly commended for my participation and the other departments received the riot act.

Richard was a teetotaler. At a hospital function, when he was the administrator, Sister flew down to attend the affair with the mother general. They were all sitting together at the same table. I stopped by to greet Sister and whispered to inquire if she would like a margarita.

Sister introduced me to the mother general and said, "Gus is buying the drinks, would you like a margarita?" The Mother General nodded yes. When I brought the drinks to the table, I whispered to Sister, "I think I am in trouble; Richard is glaring at me."

She smilingly whispered, "Thanks Gus, and don't worry about him."

Richard's private secretary Linda and I were very close friends. We enjoyed going out to dinner after work and always had a lot of fun together. Linda was mischievous by nature and loved being involved in many of our administrative antics as an initiator or being very participatory. Linda attended the same church as Richard and their congregation could be described as teetotalers. While at the hospital, Linda had a minor hospitalization. When greeting her mother and some of the ladies from their church, I made a faux pas. I said, "Linda is feeling great—she's thirsty for a margarita." Linda laughingly reprimanded me for opening my big mouth to the disdainful church teetotalers.

We had a patient who was quite seriously ill and I was working with her daughter on the financial issues. She was extremely attractive and very cooperative in addressing her mother's needs.

On one occasion, the admitting manager Martha (a.k.a. Auntie Mame) stopped by my office after the patient's daughter had finished meeting with me.

"Gus, I could sense fireworks between the two of you, like an instant attraction."

"No, Martha, there is no attraction, besides it would be unprofessional to start dating the daughter of a patient."

"Gus, I could see the fireworks between the two of you."

"No!"

The daughter was living in a newly acquired home, which she was refurbishing. And she had purchased a large brass bed from a store near Martha's home. Martha had admired the same bed and noticed a sold ticket on it in the daughter's name. While it was coincidental, it was a small community at the time.

A few weeks later, I found myself in that beautiful brass bed and I pensively and smilingly thought to myself, "If Martha could only see me now."

My entrance into the daughter's life came in the aftermath of her ending a long-term relationship. It was nothing more than a brief fling for both of us, but a very pleasant sojourn.

When I arrived in Ventura, I took tennis lessons to improve my game. Fortunately, I had a great tennis instructor who was many years younger than I. He was full of fun, single, and a real Casanova. He had befriended the dean of the Ventura School of Law, who, along with leasing the school building, had also acquired the use of four tennis courts. The facility had formerly been a Catholic private school, and it had been converted to a retirement home for the sisters.

My tennis partner personally resurfaced the two top tennis courts for teaching lessons and for our private use. Also, the lower two courts were available to the law students or whomever, based on the tennis instructor's discretion. Normally, the two upper courts kept us totally occupied throughout the daylight hours.

The dean had a heavy teaching and administrative schedule. He was a good tennis player, and he really enjoyed being able to get on the courts. He was basically a very private person with an air of aloofness—until you got to know him.

Permission to use the courts was on his terms. I took lessons from my instructor for some time, and then we just became friends and tennis buddies. The dean would join us and one day said, "Gus, your instructor and I both have keys to the tennis courts and here is yours." I had arrived! The dean and I started playing tennis each week regularly thereafter. Later, the dean asked if I would be interested in attending law classes. I declined, informing him that I had taken several units of law over the years and probably couldn't list the elements of a contract.

The dean also had a law school in Santa Barbara. During that period, every one of his qualifying students that year had passed the bar examination. He received an abundant share of accolades. We had the tennis courts for over ten years, until a new law school building was constructed elsewhere. In that setting, it was a wonderful time and place as we had so much fun.

All of the women loved my tennis pal. To accommodate his private life, he had the use of a small mobile unit that was parked just below the tennis courts. The dean owned the mobile unit, but my pal would occasionally spend the night there. One morning he and a lady friend were feeling very amorous and suddenly, during their physical activities, the lady surprisingly said, "I think this unit is moving!" He jumped up and opened the door to find a truck towing the mobile unit—fulfilling an order from the dean. When he told us the story, we laughed for days. When referring to him my friends would say, "That guy—the one with the mobile unit that moves unpredictably!"

The tennis pro had many friends who were great tennis players and who would frequent the courts. He would schedule his tennis hours for his own personal use between lessons. A tennis player acquaintance of my tennis pal was a writer who took the game extremely seriously. He was both obnoxious and truculent when the circumstances during a tennis match were not in his favor—and he freely expressed his temerity. His performance dictated his volatile mood swings. This individual casually dropped by one day for a possible game. One of my tennis pal's personal friends was in town, and he stopped by the courts. The visiting friend was an excellent minor-league baseball player. He also had a brother on one of the major leagues—a well-known celebrity star. The friend was an all-round athlete, but frankly had played very little tennis. He was not too keen on individual sports—preferring group participation sports. The obstreperous tennis player (the writer) asked the visiting friend, "Would you like to play a set of tennis with me?"

"I am a fairly good athlete, but I must caution you, I am no tennis player."

"No problem, let's just play it by ear."

Mr. Casanova and I were rallying on the second court. I said, sotto voce, "Suppose your baseball buddy wins the set?" We exchanged glances.

For the sake of brevity, I'll just say that the novice won and his opponent departed screaming and yelling! The victor was in total bewilderment that his opponent's behavior lacked such gamesmanship, and he looked at the two of us in puzzlement as we screamed hysterically.

When we calmed down, we explained why we were so delighted. We also explained that his opponent's erratic behavior was always prevalent when he lost a match.

Several of my female employees were involved in women's groups in both Ventura and Oxnard. Through their instigation and my involvement with these groups, I received Boss of the Year awards on two occasions. One was from the American Businesswomen's Association; the other from the Oxnard Credit Women's Association.

The Sisters of Mercy started presenting special awards each year to persons who had exemplified the mission of the Sisters of Mercy. More than one person can be selected each year, and the selection process includes persons in the organization and in the community as well. The first-year recipient from our hospital was an outstanding social worker in our hospice program. She had been instrumental in enhancing our community outreach program and was very deserving of the award. The second year was forthcoming and I received an invitation to the dinner. I went to my boss and asked if I could be excused as I had been involved in so many activities and didn't want to attend. He said, "You will have fun. It is a nice event. Bring a date and sit with me and my wife."

The evening of the affair, my date Betty and I went to our favorite Mexican restaurant and had a margarita before proceeding to the event. She also worked at the hospital and said,

"Why don't we just stay here and have dinner and stop by later?"

I said, "No, let's go now."

The TV personality Wink Martindale's daughter worked in our community relations department and greeted me at the door as I arrived. She said, "It's about time you got here, Gus."

I thought her comment was somewhat strange, but proceeded with Betty to the banquet room. One of the sisters, who was a friend said, "Gus, I have an extra boutonniere." She pinned it onto my lapel as she greeted me at the door. I thought that was a kind gesture and my date and I headed for the bar.

I glanced across the room and saw a lady who looked like my sister Marjorie, but thought no more of it. Suddenly, I saw my two nieces in front of me, followed by several of our sisters forming a semi circle around me and smiling at me. "What is going on?"

They all laughed and I then surmised I was to be one of the honorees.

It was great having Richard attend and my favorite sister from the Mother House also attended. Seeing Sister simply added to the anticipation of a great evening. During the dinner, with Betty and family at a single table, Betty kept saying, "You had better think up a thank you speech right away, what are you going to say?"

My niece Robin said, "Don't worry about Uncle Gus. He's resourceful; he'll think of something."

I went gangster on a couple of incidents: "The infamous St. Valentine's Massacre actually took place at this hospital when I sent a valentine to Sister and signed the CFO's name."

My admitting manager, Martha, and her husband were sitting close by. I pointed to her and said, "We are the Bonnie and Clyde at the hospital. I drive her to the local Medi-Cal office to pick-up our authorizations for billing. She runs in and picks up the cards and I remain in the car with the motor running."

I presented both incidents with embellishments that apparently warranted a wild ovation, and I thanked the sisters for their generous recognition. A prominent member of the community also received the same award and Sister thanked him graciously for his service.

In response to my St. Valentine's story and recognition Sister said, "I want to assure everyone that I am still very much aware of Gus's mischievous tendencies, which undisputedly require my further guidance."

Poor Richard had laryngitis that evening, but managed to say, "Every time I turn around you are being honored by someone—I have never received one award since I have been here."

Here is my message to Richard: You became the first lay administrator at SJRMC. You were young and respected by all. You are blessed with a wonderful family and a fabulous salary to boot. And you have a great sense of humor, too. You have it all.

The hospital was fortunate to recruit a wonderful public relations specialist, Karen. She was remarkable with print media, preparing brochures and handouts and other documentation that I needed when conducting workshops and other promotional events. She was gifted and had an effervescent manner, and freely expressed new ideas in promotional planning and executing them so proficiently. She had an octopus-type of behavior in fulfilling her objectives—total involvement was her hallmark. She stopped by my office one morning and said, "Gus, the employee awards dinner is coming up shortly. This year I am planning an Academy Awards theme! How does that sound to you?"

"Sounds great and fun."

"I want you to co-host with me the entire evening."

"Okay, with the proviso that you accept the leadership role in this duet."

"No problem, Gus. I thought we would interview the awardees as they arrive. We'll work together, along with a cameraman. After the cocktail period and dinner we'll unite again and start the presentations."

"Do you want me to be, as they say, 'prim and proper,' or do you want me to just be myself?"

"Just be Gus! I'll prepare the awards list and we can make the presentations in tandem. You know the awardees so much better than I, so put forth your humorous comments and applicable one-liners, which you do so well, to personalize each of the awardees."

"Tasteful, but fun, right!"

"Exactly!"

Thanks to her great planning, it was a magical evening. It was one of my most favorite events.

Also attending was a visiting Sister of Mercy, who was working toward her Ph.D. A few days before the ceremony, Sister had spent several hours with me discussing the practical applications that coincided with her theoretical studies. My role was to espouse my thoughts, impressions, and experiences in healthcare that she wanted to incorporate conjunctively in her thesis. Complimentarily, she took copious notes.

Toward the end of the evening, and after I left the dance floor with my date, Sister pulled me aside. "Well, Mr. Popularity, how about buying this friend an after-dinner drink and engaging in a little conversation?"

"I'm with you, Sister."

"And, by the way, Gus, your performance this evening was outstanding."

Karen and Sister were two remarkable ladies in their own fields. Both women were extremely intelligent, gracious, and well versed. I had a sponge-like attitude in being with outstanding persons; I attempted to absorb their great qualities. I recall that old maxim: You are judged by the company you keep.

I was blessed with a good staff and we worked well together and very much like a family. During one particular period, a couple of my employees had certain family obligations, which meant that they wanted to change their working hours to accommodate those personal needs.

I pulled the entire department together and discussed the problem. I said, "Our salaries are based on a schedule over which I have no control; however, I would like to accommodate our people when they need to fulfill certain obligations apart from work. If any of you would like to change your hours to accommodate family or home interests, let me know. Also, bear in mind that I am placing myself fully responsible for this off-of the-wall proposal, but my trust is with each and every one of you. In the process, we must be fully staffed to accommodate our breaks and lunch hours."

Two women who had requested special temporary hour changes received approval. A third woman requested to join two hardworking trustworthy employees on the evening shift, which I also approved. Later, the two evening persons, however, informed the third that she was not pulling her weight in the evenings and needed to return to the day shift. Sometimes conscientious and diligent employees solve the problem. Done!

One of those two women had Crohn's disease. I used to tell the staff—not in her presence—that if we had her condition and felt the way she felt on her best day, we would all be home ill in bed. She was the most organized person I had ever met. She would have files in process, files needing this or that, and she typed with two fingers. No one came close to her individual daily output. Everyone loved her and admitted that she had no competition. She was blessed with both agility and an organized mind.

Our people really worked hard and, occasionally, we would have a potluck luncheon in the business office. We would have our admitting and our ancillary units join us. I would also occasionally do something special in the early morning for breakfast by bringing fruit, rolls, and doughnuts to the department. As I had fifty-five employees, at Christmastime I would go to our gift shop and select about eight gifts, such as crystal pieces, china, or quality items, and have them gift wrapped. Everyone would place his or her name in a hat and we would have eight persons draw a name. This plan worked out very well—as the gifts were quality items and the recipients were appreciative. Those who didn't win a gift would say, "Maybe next year" or "I won last year." All agreed it was done fairly.

One of my employees stopped by my office to tell me a confidential situation. A day or so later she came to see me very disgruntled and asked, "Why did you disregard my confidentiality and pass that information on to another person?"

I said, "Other than me, who else did you tell?"

She said, "I told one of my co-workers, who is my friend. She would never tell anyone."

I responded by saying, "I told no one."

A day or so later she stopped by and said very nonchalantly, "I just learned that it was my friend who told the other person." She avoided any apology to me.

I replied, "Never again tell me any of your confidential information. I don't want to hear it." Situations such as being wrongly accused bring out the worst of my Scorpio birth month personality. (Reminiscent of that stolen pen at school.)

Conversely, another one of my employees stopped by to see me. Apparently, she had some personal problems that she had discussed with a couple of her co-workers. They both informed her that she should stop by and discuss her situation with me. They went on to say that I could be helpful to her and that I was trustworthy and extremely discreet regarding confidentiality. She informed me of the facts, and I assured her that her family member's problems were unrelated to her.

As time passed, I expressed my thoughts to her. After he, the family member, had gone through continuous professional counseling, she realized that I had nailed the problem on the head. She could not believe that I had such insight. I said, "After a while it becomes easy."

Sometime later, she and her husband and I attended the same function. She beamed at me throughout the evening in appreciation for my support in helping her through a very difficult family situation. However, I learned that it is important to know when and—more importantly—when not to become involved in personal situations relating to employees.

My niece Robin became interested in the healthcare field. One Sunday, I was at her family home in Woodland Hills. The house and pool and recreational area were loaded with family and friends—a normal weekend.

She and I took her University of California catalog and seated ourselves on the diving board for privacy to review the courses for healthcare. Because of my years in healthcare, I knew of some of the professors at the university in the program. The program addressed the need to work in a healthcare setting as part of the overall educational program. I suggested she fulfill her onsite requisites at SJRMC. I further suggested that she should report to our admitting and patient representative manager, Martha. She would be certain to provide Robin with both sufficient and excellent training.

When the plan was finally under way, I really enjoyed Robin coming to the hospital each week and working with our patient representatives. She soon became extremely proficient in performing her assigned duties.

She worked as an unpaid intern, but was a true team player, as she worked with each patient representative. Robin, with alacrity, would pick-up any slack or overload when needed. Needless to say, she pleased me tremendously. At the end of each day, she would stop by my office. If I was available, I would walk her to her car.

I truly enjoyed having her at my workplace, and I was really pleased with her performance. She was gracious to our patients and popular among her co-workers. She and I were both intended for service in the healthcare field.

Before Robin's graduation, one of her instructors was to make a fieldtrip to our hospital for an assessment of the duties she performed at the hospital. The onsite review was a portion of her final grades. A meeting was arranged with her instructor, and Martha and I were in my office with Robin awaiting his arrival. Robin said, "Uncle Gus, don't tell my instructor that we are family!"

I replied, "Are you concerned about nepotism?"

"Yes!"

When her instructor arrived, and after the amenities, I said, "Robin is my niece. Both Martha and I are what would be considered bread-and-butter people. In other words, we are working in the trenches along with our employees." I further stated that it behooved us to be certain that Robin received the best possible training. Our work plan included an overall understanding of the functions within the admitting office, as well as the patient accounts department.

The instructor said, "Robin, you are a very fortunate student to be in such favorable surroundings and to receive such personal attention in the process. I like the 'bread-and-butter' approach of being in the trenches and learning all phases of the business."

With the help of Martha and me, Robin came through with flying colors and very much deserved the good report card she received from us. The instructor was a very down-to-earth person and he was obviously pleased with our meeting. Robin brushed aside my spilling of the beans about our relationship.

Robin had attended Pierce Junior College, spent a year at Pepperdine, and attended California State University at Northridge for four years. She graduated with a bachelor of science in health administration.

Upon completion of Robin's studies, Martha stopped by my office and said, "Gus, I want to hire Robin as a patient representative for an unspecified period of time."

"Absolutely no!"

"Why?"

"Martha, there are several other employees that view that position as a step upwards and would like the opportunity to apply."

"Robin is fully trained, well-liked and respected, and no one would resent her accepting that position."

"No!"

"Gus, I want Robin and I am going over your head if necessary to bring her onboard. Your choice."

"No!"

Martha proceeded and met with the CFO, "I want you to sign this form so that I can hire Robin as a patient representative for an unspecified period of time."

"Martha, where does Gus stand on this?"

"Forget him, just sign the form. I have everything under control." He signed the form.

Robin returned to work as a paid employee. Virtually every single person in the department stopped by my office to tell me how pleased they were at having Robin return to work as an employee.

Martha was victorious when I requested a very small slice of humble pie!

At SJRMC we had a happy family atmosphere among our departmental employees and freely expressed our opinions. Gayle, our senior patient representative and my first hire, befriended Robin from day one. Gayle was a very devoted and an excellent employee, but slightly critical, and thought I was somewhat demanding in my expectations for the department. Behind my back, Gayle and others referred to me as "Father." One day Gayle said to Robin, "He is so demanding at times—always seeking perfection."

Robin quickly responded, "Gayle, how would you like him for an uncle?" Robin was always right down the middle—one of the gang—and they loved her.

Exactly a year to the day after I was presented with the Mercy Award, I attended the same function. I returned home to find a letter from my unknown Munro relatives in Ontario, Canada. I was so surprised and excited to hear from them that I telephoned them the following day. They had tracked me down through one of my first cousins. Frankly, this had been our first contact. I had known that they were in Ontario, but knew nothing about them. The original Scottish settlers had come to Canada and settled in one of three locations: Nova Scotia, southern Ontario, and Selkirk, Manitoba. Our Munro clan had chosen Ontario.

I was truly excited to hear from them, and it was absolutely shocking to me. I immediately made arrangements to take my seventeen-year-old niece, Michele (Robin's sister) with me to visit our "long lost" Munro relatives in Eastern Canada.

I received a telephone call a day or so before leaving on our trip. Jack, the son of the CFO I had worked under at The Hospital of the Good Samaritan, sadly informed me that his mother had passed away. I was shocked, as she was still a middle-aged person. Unfortunately, she had had a serious illness. After expressing my condolences, he asked if I would like be a pallbearer at his mother's funeral. I informed him that I was leaving for eastern Canada and would be unable to attend. He clearly understood my situation. "Mr. Munro, my mother believed you were one of the nicest men she had known. She further stated that you were excellent in fulfilling all of your responsibilities at the hospital and that you had wonderful qualities as a human being."

"Jack, coming from your mother, that is a tremendous compliment."

"Mr. Munro, you are the first person I have called. That should attest to those compliments. My mother had tremendous respect for you and also considered you to be an example to others as a standard."

I mentioned that, when I had told his mother that I was leaving that hospital, she simply cried openly and I had quietly left her office. This had been a very profound experience and I had never previously encountered anything like it. Somewhat surprised, right after leaving her office I had stopped by to see a nursing administrator and explained the situation. Our thoughts were sympathetically directed to the CFO. I asked that she provide a letter of reference to me. She was the one that informed me that I was to be honored as employee of the year, which I discussed earlier.

Jack's grandfather had been the brew master at the Anheuser Busch Brewery in St. Louis for many years. While in college, Jack's mother had been a straight-A student and breezed through obtaining her CPA. Their lineage was that of a solid American family, and Jack shared his mother's great qualities, as did his sister. I have been blessed in having been associated with fine outstanding individuals such as his mother. It was very consoling to me to receive such recognition from her after her departure from this earth.

17

Aside from receiving such sad news, Michele and I were very excited to meet our relatives in eastern Canada. We were both very interested in our Munro history. The Munro ownership of our original Ontario property dated back to about 1830, and was currently under the stewardship of Ray Munro, who was a first cousin to my father. He was, however, over twenty years younger than my father was—a different generation. Ray and his wife Dorothy were the parents of one son and three daughters, all married with children. Their son and his family resided on the same property.

Upon our arrival, Ray and a couple of family members met us at the airport in Toronto. Before proceeding to their home, they stopped at a small Scottish Presbyterian church. A graveyard was adjacent to the property. We learned that many of our relatives, including the original ancestors, had been buried there. Michele took pictures of the church and tombstones for posterity.

From there we stopped at their home for lunch and had a quick tour of their properties. Michele and I were soon to learn that their farmland was breathtakingly beautiful with fields, grazing meadows, wooded areas, and lakes.

The original settlers' home was a wood-frame structure. It remains in semi-ruin on the property. Ray and Dorothy were true workaholics and their days were long and very hard. He mentioned that one day he would like to restore the original settlers' home, but currently they had a full schedule.

What surprised me the most was the fact that they had over two hundred head of Murray Grey beef cattle. I hadn't realized that southern Ontario was cattle country.

I learned that movie companies liked filming on their property. *An Incident in a Small Town*, which starred Walter Matthau, Henry Morgan, and Stephanie Zimbalist, was filmed on their farmlands. One prominent Hollywood character actor actually pleaded with my cousin to sell him at least one acre of their land for his own use. Being a traditionalist, my cousin declined his offer.

I had arranged motel accommodations in town, as we did not really know our relatives. We ended the day visiting other cousins and one whose wife had just baked some fruitcake, which I love. It was delicious.

She enters her fruitcake each year at their local fair, and she always is awarded the second prize. I said that she was going to win first prize this year as it was outstanding. Michele, at that time, was a very picky eater, but curiosity got the better of her and she decided to try the fruitcake. She took one bite and, with a look of utter revulsion, handed the remaining fruitcake to me, as if it were a dead, smelly fish. It was, unfortunately, an Academy Award performance. I said to myself, *Just wait till we get to the motel. Here I am trying to ingratiate myself with these cousins I just barely met!*

We said good night to our family that evening, after spending the day meeting all of our relatives, seeing the landscape, and learning the history at the church. We had had so much to talk about. Michele and I had never ever had an argument. As soon as we entered the motel alone, I said in a reprimanding way, "I cannot believe you and that fruitcake incident." Our eyes quickly met and we started to laugh. We were near hysteria. The following morning, I got up early to go for a run and, when I returned to the motel, we just looked at each other and started cracking up again. We knew our relatives would be picking us up shortly for breakfast and I said that we must learn to control ourselves.

The next couple of days we went sightseeing in Toronto and to visit some local gardens and other points of interest. One of my first cousins, whom I hadn't seen since I was about fifteen, was en route from northern Ontario with his wife and daughter to join us. That morning, we had visited with a cousin who was a registered nurse at the local hospital. I informed her that I would like to stop by and see their facility before we returned to California.

That afternoon, Ray decided to provide a little tour of their farmland. Ray and Dorothy were both teetotalers. However, the prior Munro generations had operated a whiskey still in the woodlands of the property. Ray wanted to include it on our tour.

Ray's grandson Daniel, age seven, got on the tractor and Ray, Michele, and I stood on a wagon attached to it. Unfortunately, it was a damp day and my sinuses were bothering me, and that affected my equilibrium. Shortly after we started our tour, I lost my balance and fell backwards off of the wagon and landed on a pile of poles.

Ray instructed Michele to go with him immediately, so that they could call the paramedics and await their arrival to guide them to the location. He instructed Daniel to remain with me. I was stretched out on those poles in horrible pain and slightly disoriented. Daniel tearfully told me, "Uncle Gus, I have to leave you before the police get here, or they'll put me in jail! This is all my fault!"

"Daniel, just stay with me until the ambulance arrives. You have done nothing wrong, I just fell on my own. Don't be upset—it's not your fault."

I arrived in the emergency room at the hospital. My registered nurse cousin had rushed and arrived simultaneously. She placed a bag over my face, as I was hyperventilating.

I managed to facetiously say to her, "This is not how I envisioned my visit to your hospital."

I was admitted to the hospital thereafter with a fractured shoulder and with a lot of trauma in my left arm.

My poor little Daniel, that first evening he was so distraught. He took his sleeping bag and placed it at the end of his parents' bed. He said, "Uncle Gus was my friend, but he will hate me now."

The next morning, his father took him to see me at the hospital to assure him all was well. Before returning home they stopped by to see the grandparents. The grandmother said to Daniel, "Poor Uncle Gus and his fractured shoulder."

Daniel replied, "Don't worry about him. He's okay and he is not mad at me anyway."

Meanwhile, Michele was having a good time getting to know several cousins her age. I gave her my wallet so that she could take the cousins to the movies and hit the local fast food places. I also instructed her to make our reservation to return home, so I could be admitted to my own hospital for further care. She was terrific and took care of all of our arrangements appropriately without question or hesitation. Unbelievable!

Before leaving the hospital for home, I did get an afternoon pass to visit with my relatives, as they were having a family reunion in our honor. Dorothy made a wonderful luncheon with my favorite, Lake Superior white fish, and it was fun getting to see all of our cousins at one location.

In the course of the afternoon, Daniel casually came over to see me sitting with my arm in a sling and doped with medication. He said, in all seriousness, "Uncle Gus, I would love to take you for one more ride before you leave." I was speechless; his comments were timed perfectly, making it the best line I ever heard. At age seven, he was just trying to be accommodating and he had no idea what a funny line he had composed. Like, yeah, all I need is another ride to finish me off!

I returned to SJRMC and, after a couple of days, the doctor decided against surgery and alternately ordered outpatient treatments in physical therapy. I had a wonderful therapist who gave me treatments daily.

At the end of the treatment plan, I mentioned that I was really grateful for her good work and I asked if I could take her to dinner to show my appreciation.

At dinner, I had the craziest idea to tell the waitress that it was my therapist's birthday. I thought, *Why am I thinking of anything so stupid?* I tried to dismiss the thought. I personally dread those surprise birthday antics—everyone coming to the table with a song, a cupcake, and candle. As we were driving back to SJRMC to her car, she informed me that it was a special day. She exclaimed, "Today is my birthday! Thank you so much for the nice evening!" (Intuition time!)

While at SJRMC I conducted many Medicare programs for the senior popula-tion in Ventura County. Several were held at the hospital, and many took place in senior communities—mainly the Oxnard area. I would explain benefits to them and to those seniors with state or federal plans that they had in place of Medicare. I discussed other supplementary plans for those with Medicare. The Sisters of Mercy, along with other hospital groups, offered a special seniors pro-gram. The program allowed certain discounts and offered some assistance to those persons with limited coverage on the supplementary plans.

The special seniors program got underway and I was totally responsible for initiating our program. Our patient representative Jean and I worked on initiat-ing the various necessary steps. We visited several senior residential and social centers located in the community. I made presentations at bingo games, potluck lunches and dinners, and other functions and, with great momentum, we signed hundreds of seniors to the program within a short period of time.

I always enjoyed participating in these gatherings to show our presence in the community. It afforded us the opportunity to get good feedback regarding our performance at the hospital. We were cognizant that these folks were our patients and we their hospital. We often brought a member from our pharmacy to discuss pharmaceutical issues, and we brought other professionals who offered topics of interest. These speakers were a successful impetus in bringing out more seniors to our sessions.

I truly enjoyed being at SJRMC. There was one brief period during which I got very upset and angry over a horrible computer conversion that really set us back. My departments had nothing to do with the debacle. I was so angry at the situation that I informed the CFO that I was going to leave. However, after a few weeks I calmed down and we diligently got everything back to normal.

This had been the second computer conversion I'd experienced. They both had gone amok and my tolerance level had reached zero. I strongly believed in a concentration of preplanning before computer conversions and/or enhancements. Those not involved in the grunt work after the conversion had a somewhat blasé attitude toward strong preliminary planning. Sometime later we were having a special management enhancement session and I asked the CFO to describe me in one word. He spontaneously replied, "Resilient!"

He further explained that I would have my down periods and then suddenly be recharged and full of enthusiasm once more without any encouragement or support from others—computer conversions being a prime example.

It was wonderful working with my CFO and our sister administrator followed by Richard over those many years. Unequivocally, SJRMC was the end of the line for me vocationally speaking. I had no desire to work anywhere else.

Unfortunately, Richard decided to move to Alaska, as he believed their educational system would be better for his growing family. Six months after he had moved to Alaska, he and his family returned to spend the Christmas holidays with relatives in Ventura. Richard stopped by my office and informed me, "Gus, I need you badly in Alaska."

"Richard, I don't think so."

"Gus, Alaska is beautiful. Anchorage is great and the hospital is state of the art. I need you badly."

"I don't think my sinus problem would be conducive to Alaska."

"Gus, it is not like Seattle or Vancouver. It is a dry cold and your sinus condition would be okay."

"Let me think about it."

"Good, I'll call you after the holidays when I return to Alaska."

Meanwhile, the CFO had accepted Richard's position as acting administrator for a short period of time before hiring a new replacement. He, himself, had been offered the promotion, but turned it down. He much preferred to remain in his current position as the CFO.

A new administrator was hired and, to put it politely, was not my cup of tea! To be certain of my immediate assessment of him, I remained another year and a half. In view of my decision, I had informed Richard that I would not be coming to Alaska. I was in a precarious position—just hating to leave SJRMC.

Not surprisingly, my first impression was lasting and I did not want to work under the new administration. I reluctantly was considering having to leave a very fulfilling life in Ventura of nearly fourteen years, leaving my nice condo, wonderful friends and associates, and a great hospital—with a family-like bonding.

I informed Robin, who had been working there for several months to move on and get another job. I wanted her reestablished elsewhere before my departure.

Quickly leaving SJRMC, Robin accepted a position at Santa Monica Hospital. Her university studies and practical working experience and the tutelage she had received with Martha and her group at SJRMC were extremely helpful in resettling in a new position. Martha had very solidly emphasized the rudimentary steps.

Robin became very responsibly involved in the admitting and patient representative areas at the new hospital. When experiencing difficult days or periods of time, she would say to Uncle Gus, pointedly and without sensitivity, "You are the one responsible for getting me started in healthcare, and it's all your fault!" (I never took umbrage.) Robin has enjoyed being in healthcare. I am proud that she has done extremely well in accepting and discharging her responsibilities—compassionately.

During my period of contemplation at SJRMC, the CFO informed me one day that they had been unsuccessful in obtaining an important renewed contract from a super major insurance company. He stated that our newly hired administrator had personally gone directly to this organization and he, too, had been denied. The CFO said that the door had been closed on our hospital and it was quite serious.

At that time I had lowered my administrative profile because of our new administrator and his regime. However, my loyalty to SJRMC ran deeply. I informed the CFO, "I can get the contract."

"Gus, if you can the hospital will be indebted to you."

I GOT IT!

One of my key persons mentioned that I never received one word of recognition; however, I was not too surprised. I was happy to be able to resolve that situation on behalf of the Sisters of Mercy who had been so kind to me.

My department managers arranged a farewell party for me at one of the old mansions in Oxnard, which was located on a military base. It was a combined birthday and farewell gathering for me. The mansion could accommodate about one hundred persons and I believe one hundred thirty-five persons wanted to attend. That really pleased me and it was a great evening. My family was included, which was the icing on the cake—thanks to my thoughtful inner circle!

My years at St. John's had been a great adventure. However, it has always been my personal commitment never to report to someone whom I do not respect.

Because of my many wonderful years at SJRMC, it was difficult to have to leave because of one person. Unfortunately, I was not alone in my thinking and personal observations that caused me to realize that I had to move on. Other persons close to me got on the same bandwagon and left. When faced with an irresolvable situation, prolonging a leave is shortsighted, indecisive, and totally unproductive—all negatives, which have had no familiarity in my personal background.

The door to Alaska was still open, and, after my many years at SJRMC, I was ready for some new excitement elsewhere. And, in the process, I would keep my options open.

18

Before I left for Alaska for my interview with Richard at Providence Hospital, I spent a day in Woodland Hills at my sister Marjorie's home. My youngest niece Michele had a boyfriend, Stephen, who was attending college and he was helping my sister to redecorate her home after classes. It was a hot October day and I had just returned home after jogging. Later that day, Michele and Stephen were to take me to the airport. I showered and put on a set of newly purchased long johns and went looking for Stephen. He was painting in the kitchen and when he saw me facetiously modeling the underwear we both started to laugh. "It is so hot today to have to wear these 'johns' to the airport and on to Anchorage."

"Why not just change into them in Alaska at the terminal?"

"Suppose the plane just lands in the field and not at the terminal?"

Michele joined us and we all laughed en route to the airport over the long johns. When I arrived at the Anchorage airport, however, I was pleased to be dressed so warmly as it was thirty-seven degrees above zero. However, I did learn that the passengers deplaned into the terminal and not onto an open field.

Richard had an evening meeting and sent one of his directors, Chet, to meet me and to take me to my hotel near Providence Hospital. Chet was in charge of the information systems at the hospital. We stopped for a nightcap and a chat, and he gave me an overall picture of the hospital and life in Alaska, which I appreciated very much. I got up at the crack of dawn and went for a walk.

When I returned Richard called and said, "Gus, I'll pick you up. Don't leave the hotel—the streets are really icy this morning."

"Sorry, your instructions are too late. I've already been combing the neighborhood."

He gave me a tour of the hospital and I met with several of his key personnel throughout the day. Richard escorted me to the business office and introduced me to their acting director Tim, who suggested we spend some time together. He was a young man and appeared very eager to exchange dialogue. "Gus, Richard has told me wonderful stories about you and I am hopeful that you will accept his offer."

"Tim, this would be a big move for me to consider; however, Richard and I have worked closely together for many years and we shall see."

"Okay, Gus. Frankly, I was thrown into this position and I don't know what the hell I'm doing. I am an internal auditor with a strong accounting background and I am totally overwhelmed being placed in this untenable position. I want you to come to Providence and bail me out. Gus, I am from the south and from a prestigious southern family. My grandfather was a U.S. Senator for years and my father a prominent civic leader in our community. And here am I in Alaska—miles away from home and deluged with work I don't understand. I'm totally lost in this situation. Help me!"

"Tim, I admire you. Based on your honesty and, at first glance, I assumed a 'southern gentleman,' too. No promises, no commitments, let's just see what happens."

"Gus, you are my last hope—please come so I can return to accounting and auditing. We have just gone through a computer conversion and we're all really overwhelmed."

I associate honesty with integrity. And it did take strength of character for Tim to open up to a complete stranger and share his inner feelings without the fear of possible repercussions.

Unbeknownst to him, he was sharing his frustrations, anxieties, and ineptness with the right person. This was a poignant experience for both of us—and paramount to my decision-making process in contemplating acceptance of the directorship being offered to me. He made a very compelling case. I could strongly relate to him, a man who had accepted a position that was unbefitting to him.

That evening Richard took several of his key personnel and me to dinner. It was a nice gesture on his part, and afforded me the opportunity to study these unfamiliar persons in a social setting. With the exception of Richard, all others ordered drinks before and some after dinner. I quietly—and hopefully inconspicuously—joined their ranks.

It was a pleasant evening and very beneficial to me in making my decision to accept Richard's proposal to join his administrative team. My thoughts regarding Tim's dilemma lingered in my mind, along with so many other considerations regarding this new position.

In selecting a new position for myself, I realized that I could never find a better person than Richard in a leadership position. He had long proven himself to me. He was a very moral, dedicated, hardworking, and decent man. And, besides that—remember—he loved my storage room, too, even after those negative comments he had made about me in casual clothes performing manual labor. His presence, in the final decision making, tipped the balance. And he eagerly wanted me to join his team.

I returned to California the following day. I accepted the position and sold my condo immediately and arranged to ship my furniture to Anchorage. These transactions all occurred in early November 1986. I purchased a nice condo, moved in, and had it redecorated before the final papers were drawn. And I leased an automobile. After about three weeks, I was totally settled in as I had a big job to fill at the hospital and no time for personal stuff.

The hospital was modern, aesthetically designed, and impressively expansive to accommodate future growth. It was the largest medical center in Alaska. The main lobby was museum like, architecturally speaking, and a nice collection of paintings adorned the hallways. I must confess that even the local moose herds were rather impressed with the structure. One morning we saw a female moose, accompanied by her two offspring, at our main entrance. They spent about an hour admiring the facility before heading back to the bush country.

The medical center operated an air service that brought patients in from all parts of Alaska. Many patients were transported from very remote small villages in the hinterland. I soon learned that our hospital was truly essential to Alaska, and we worked very closely with elected officials in Juneau on various healthcare issues. We actually had a specific administrative department in the hospital that addressed both state and federal governmental mutual issues and concerns.

Shortly after joining the hospital, I found myself working with our state representatives in Juneau and Washington DC. We were involved with native affairs pertaining to the welfare of both the Native American Indian and Eskimo populations and we worked closely with the Veterans Administration and the military facilities as well.

We also had to provide full services for indigent patients. As there were no county medical facilities in that state, private hospitals were required to accommodate the total population. I also privately worked directly with families in the Russian community to afford them medical assistance. The Russians proudly retained their early native culture, costumes, and picturesque fishing villages. They were interesting people, but appeared to me somewhat remote. I believe they remained within their own community to preserve their interests and culture.

I attended many meetings my first several weeks at Providence for both orientation and networking. I attended them with the proviso that someone would stop by my office and take me to and from meetings. The complex was so large it took me weeks to feel comfortable getting around on my own. In my early days I got lost several times.

The real estate lady who had helped me find my condo in Alaska stopped by the hospital with her father to join me for lunch one day. Her father was a professor at the University of Alaska and he was in a wheelchair. I met and greeted them at the main entrance and proceeded to wheel the father to our premium coffee shop. When passing through the halls, several individuals stopped me briefly regarding meetings or current issues. When the three of us arrived at our table for lunch, the father said pointedly, "I cannot believe you have just been in this hospital for a few weeks, you seem to know more people in Anchorage than I."

One evening the daughter and I went to a very popular and unique Quonset hut restaurant for dinner. Upon arrival, she excused herself. Due to the compactness of the structure, people were seated quite close together and I immediately started engaging in a conversation with one of the daily newspaper writers and his wife, who were sitting close by. When my date returned I introduced her and she said later, "One cannot leave you for three minutes—you are so engaging. Everyone is drawn to you." Ironically, I had been told, but never experienced, that many Alaskans are somewhat aloof and reserved until they get to know you.

Many of the sisters based at the hospital were from the Province of Quebec, which I found interesting. Their predecessors had journeyed to Alaska in the early territorial days to address the needs of the early settlers and the native and nomadic population. Unfortunately, in conversing with the sister in charge of the order, I made mention, as a former Canadian from British Columbia, that I hoped Quebec would remain within the Canadian union and not become independent. She disliked me from the time I made that comment, and the feeling was mutual. I had always had great relationships with sisters and she was definitely the exception.

My childhood ties with members of a large French Canadian family ran deeply, as they had become, emotionally, part of my own family. I had had close kinships with other friends from Quebec. Frankly, while I vehemently disagreed, I did respect her personal opinion in wishing a separate Quebec. However, it was her truculent response to my divergent opinion that ticked me off. She practiced rigidity in other areas, too.

Richard was really happy to have me onboard. When he left SJRMC he requested of his new Alaskan employer not to be named the administrator, but rather the chief operating officer (COO) or the chief financial officer (CFO) or both. He preferred COO, as he would be responsible for running the hospital on a day-to-day basis. He immediately informed me that I would play a key role in his inner administrative circle. One of his most pressing needs was to help create better relationships with the medical staff. I assured him that I would do my best.

I met one of Richard's close friends, an Anchorage businessman and a member of his church, who privately informed me that he and Richard had traveled to Seattle on business and had had a lengthy conversation about me during the flight. Richard said that he and I had worked closely together at SJRMC and thought I did a great job for the hospital. He said that he didn't realize how good I was until he reached Alaska. Richard informed him that I had been absolutely outstanding, but he had never realized the extent until he started interacting with the folks in this Alaskan hospital. He said he would give his right arm to get me up there. Nice comments for a dropout to receive and from one so pragmatically oriented.

With my rotten luck, combined with my seemingly perennial involvement with Murphy and his law, I learned that the hospital had just experienced a major computer installation with a leading provider. Fortunately, I was familiar with their system. Additionally, the key installation specialist, Beverly, had installed our system years earlier at SJRMC. Beverly was working out of the Seattle office of her company, so I waited with great anticipation for her next visit to rekindle our relationship and to discuss mutual concerns. To make a long story short, after several months, Beverly came onboard and became my assistant director of admissions and business services. Her knowledge of our newly installed computer system was definitely an enhancement for us.

Because of the conversion and many other very basic procedures and other factors that had been somewhat overlooked, I was totally overwhelmed with work. Beverly, before starting at the hospital, had focused on refining the systems on her onsite visits. I worked long hours trying to bring our accounts receivable to a manageable level. Due to the conversion, all data had to be reentered into the system, which was a very lengthy and laborious process. It also entailed numerous basic audits to be certain we had total accountability in working our open accounts.

I worked every single day—at the very least sixty hours every week—to get all of my departments functioning at acceptable levels. I loathed having loose ends that could be subject to criticism—they were nightmarish and untenable and foreign to my personal expectations.

Along with problems relating to the accounts receivable and the need to refine the new computer system, I had multiple staff problems—supervisor versus employee sort of problems. I met regularly with my staff and informed them that I had an open-door policy and told them they should feel free to see me at any time. One employee came to my office three times just to confirm that I said I had an open door policy. That incident brought forth a series of meetings that were well attended and during which issues were very candidly discussed. Those meetings turned out to be very constructive and cleared the air on various issues. However, my work was really cut out for me, and I felt somewhat overwhelmed.

Many areas needed immediate attention, motivation, and guidance as we reinvented wheels to get the operation running on a sound basis. I had to set a standard of being tenacious, consistent, and a good team player, working with my staff to get things accomplished. To begin with, just getting the troops moving in the right direction was an arduous task. Many looked at me thinking I would work hard for a while, then either leave or slacken off as some of my predecessors seemed to have done. They didn't know me—I set a standard and maintained it.

Each weekend I would have a crew working with me in the business office. One employee, Marilyn, was sitting at her desk late Saturday afternoon in tears. I approached her questioningly and with concern, "Why are you so upset? Have I offended you?"

She said, very mild mannerly and somewhat hesitantly, "I am so embarrassed and feel foolish as you are telling us to get back to the basics, and everything you say makes perfect sense."

"Marilyn, we just simply need to roll up our sleeves and get the department up to date and maintain it accordingly."

"May I work extra time to assist in achieving our goals?"

"Yes!"

"Mr. Munro, I really appreciate being able to help in this project." She and I started working together every weekend—sometimes with other employees helping out, too.

After a few weeks, Marilyn informed me that she had been disgruntled sometime before my arrival and had been thinking of transferring out of the business office. There was a prominent psychic residing in Anchorage and she had sought her help. The psychic informed her that a new director would come onboard and would be sympathetic to her concerns. She told Marilyn to make no change and to await his arrival.

Marilyn further stated that the psychic had been involved in offering her services to legal authorities. The unfortunate aftermath was that she became a victim when someone shot her in the face. Apparently, she had been providing the legal authorities sound information; fortunately, she recovered, but soon after left Anchorage to protect her safety.

Marilyn said that the psychic had given her tremendous insight, and she was sorry for her departure, but understood the safety factor. Marilyn had a nice family and her son came to work with us part-time after school and full-time during the summer months. He worked as a concierge in our admitting office and he would work extra hours on the weekends to help us with accounts receivable. Marilyn and I would work projects all weekend relating to our accounts receivable. She would carry on during the week to complete the work, and we would start over again the following Saturday with the next section—an ongoing process.

I am so thankful to have known them, as we all worked so diligently in getting everything up to date. We three really bonded, and, while I was there, I considered them my Alaska family. I absolutely adored them.

This family was part Native, and I taught Marilyn's grandson (age three) my version of the Ketchikan Indian Rain Dance. Marilyn's family was from there. And she would get hysterical watching us perform. She said she wished that her beloved grandmother, who was departed, could have seen me perform the Ketchikan Indian Rain Dance with her grandson. She would have loved it.

Now, here is another story about her precocious grandson: Marilyn spent most of her free time with her grandson, whom she absolutely adored. One day she picked him up from home and brought him to her house to spend the weekend. On arriving at Marilyn's house, the grandson muttered something to her about turning on the lights. She inquired, "What did you say about turning on the lights?"

He repeated "Turn on the f—-ing lights!"

Shocked she quickly grabbed him and took him into the bathroom. She impulsively thought to wash his mouth with soap, but decided to interrogate him. She said, "Who taught you that bad language?"

He nonchalantly said, "It was the baby sitter wanting the lights on because her boyfriend was coming over."

Marilyn kept repeating to her grandson not to use those bad words.

Sometime later a family member passed away and Marilyn's son conducted the memorial service—he was only near nineteen, but his performance was magnificent. Meanwhile, said grandson was sitting or lying on my lap during the total service. Suddenly he looked upward at the ceiling and said, "Gus, look at all of those f—-ing lights."

One of my managers was sitting next to us; she was a close friend to Marilyn. After the grandson's comments, she and I looked at each other and both, almost in states of convulsion, tried to retain our composure. We were, after all, at a funeral service. After the service that friend and I went ballistic. She had heard the original story long before the service, so this had been the proverbial (foul-mouthed!) icing on the cake. In all fairness, apart from the F-word, the grandson was a cute little guy and we adored him and his antics. (I hate the F-word.)

Marilyn's son had been in a slight accident with her car and it had required some minor repairs. There had been a slight bone of contention, as he had claimed to have been misdirected or instructed by his passenger, his twin sister. However, her son was very sensitive and a little embarrassed about the incident, as he was a very cautious driver. He was quite unhappy.

I stopped over to their house one night and Marilyn's grandson brought his toy car to me. It was in two pieces. I picked up the two parts and said, to add levity, "Well, it looks like your uncle has been driving your car, too."

Marilyn roared along with said son—and that seemed to take the edge off of things regarding the auto accident. A humorous gesture can bring forth harmony.

I did spend a lot of time with this family—many hours, of course, at work, and we did go out for dinners. Both mother and son loved to go to weekly bingo games. They were very lucky and usually won something each week. I joined them on a couple of occasions and it was clear to both of them that bingo was not my forte. They individually played several cards and I about four. Mother or son had to check my cards constantly, as I lacked focus. I missed numbers and won and didn't know it. Fortunately, they would find my win in time to call. Based on their alertness, I gave them my winnings; however, they rejoiced when I stopped playing bingo.

I was very grateful to Chet for greeting me at the airport on my first trip to Anchorage and getting me settled that first night. Chet's life partner was a registered nurse and in charge of a newly formed rehabilitation services unit. Unfortunately, being a new department, they ran into some problems on reimbursement through an intermediary and the situation was in limbo when I arrived. Several claims were involved and represented a substantial amount of money. The difficult problem had been set on a back burner, but it still was a contentious topic.

I wanted to express my gratitude for Chet's kindness in welcoming me by giving this unresolved issue my immediate attention. Additionally, it was ultimately my responsibility to resolve the situation expeditiously. Working with the key persons at the intermediary's office, we finally received payment on every unpaid claim at the scheduled rate of reimbursement. As a new director working with new intermediaries, I felt victorious in getting that situation amicably resolved. It had been a serious bone of contention for the rehabilitation services unit as well as for Richard and his administrative team.

Unfortunately, when I resolved the issues and got the outstanding claims paid, Chet's partner, who was in charge of rehab services, viewed my participation negatively. She stopped by to see me and said, "Well, we did all of the work, and you get the credit."

"No, I did my job to see that we were reimbursed for the good services you provided your patients."

"Yeah, yeah, Gus."

Suddenly and sadly, Chet took seriously ill. He was in his thirties. During his illness, I sat next to his lady at a staff meeting, took her hand, and said that I prayed morning and night for Chet's recovery. She kept looking at me throughout the meeting, and that started a better rapport for us from that day forth. Sadly, this remarkable young man, loaded with fine qualities and talent, passed away several weeks later. His lady was truly a wonderful person—so dedicated—but devastated over his unexpected death. It was so sad for her and all to endure.

I had another similar experience. Our information systems unit provided a special representative for each department and/or set of departments, to work with them in meeting their daily needs and objectives. I was fortunate to have a young lady in her early thirties as my special information systems representative. She was a registered nurse, but decided on using her medical training skills in a hospital setting in information systems. She was great to work with and, after working together with me for some time, she arranged a special private meeting.

She told me how much she enjoyed working with me and that she had great respect for the way I effectively managed my departments. She further stated that I was not an information systems type person and I relied heavily on her input and expertise—which was all very true. She said that we made a great team and she wanted me to be included in her future plans. Unfortunately, I never had the opportunity to meet her husband while we were formulating those plans.

Her husband was in his early thirties and he was a squadron leader in the air force. Apparently, he was quite outstanding, as he was working closely with the then Soviet air force stationed on the Soviet side of the Bering Sea to be certain that no mishaps occurred while the two countries flew separate maneuvers. From all reports, they were an ideal couple and very proficient in their careers.

They had no children and her husband was planning to leave the service several months down the road. They were planning to move to Atlanta where he would become a commercial pilot. I believe that overtures had been made to a commercial airline anticipating his return to civilian life.

She attempted to convincingly appeal to me by saying, "When our plans materialize, would you consider joining us if I can find a position for myself in a medical center and one for you, too?"

"I would consider anything down the road, as I am single, getting older, and am free to move, providing my sinus condition could cope with what I assume would be a humid climate in Atlanta." This was just a spur-of-the-moment, off-of-the-top comment.

"Gus, I know the hospital field and you are not a run-of-the-mill person in this industry. We could compliment each other in seeking joint positions."

I realized that this situation, if it materialized, would be sometime down the road.

One day, I met the CFO in the hall and informed him, "I'm feeling ill. I probably have a touch of influenza. I'm heading home to rest."

He said, "Let me walk you to your car, as I have some bad news to tell you. The pilot husband of your colleague in information systems has been out on a practice mission and he is missing. It seems that all other pilots have returned safely to the base except him."

"Oh, my God!"

He continued, "Presently, a search party is out looking for him and the situation looks grim."

I rushed home in constant prayer and went to bed, glued to my radio. About an hour or so later, it was announced that his plane had been spotted, crashed into a mountainside, and he had been presumably instantaneously killed.

It was so sad. All of the wonderful attributes that I had heard of this young pilot were affirmatively echoed at his memorial service. His grieving widow left Alaska shortly thereafter and I sincerely hope she eventually found happiness.

When I first moved to Anchorage, I soon realized that the population consisted of a very participatory citizenry who used the services of their very powerful print media. Disgruntled patients would send letters to the local newspaper advocates complaining about our hospital and, particularly, about patient accounts. I took these letters seriously and took it upon myself to directly contact the patients and personally resolve their situations. On one occasion—actually my first—I personally went to the unhappy patient's office along with the supervisor involved in the incident to apologize to him. After meeting both of us and hearing our explanation of our challenges within the office, he sincerely appreciated our visit and apology.

I also worked with the newspaper advocates in the process of resolution. Fortunately, with concerted efforts we got the situation under control, and my name was used as the contact person, which, thankfully, helped in the process of stemming the tide. Complaints are nightmarish to me, especially when drawn through the media. I am grateful that Alaska was the only place I ever experienced media intervention. I am exceedingly strong on patient relations, and that has been manifested over the years by patients, their family members, and their physicians and office staff and others.

19

There was a young man, George, who hailed from Indiana, who worked in one of my departments. From viewing distance, I perceived that he and a young lady, as they sat next to one another, appeared to be spending valuable time on personal conversation. I calmly and quietly joined them by leaning over between their desks and requesting they stop chatting and continue with their work assignments. The young lady took umbrage and denied my observation.

George, apologetically, said, "Sorry, Mr. Munro," and returned to work.

When minor incidents such as this occur, I normally have a follow-up discussion, privately, with each person involved. Reexamining an incident later usually provides more of a conciliatory atmosphere for reconciliation if bad or hurt feelings remain. I met with the young lady and we ironed out our differences. She was a very good employee, extremely sensitive. A revisit of the situation helped clear the air and provided her an opportunity to air her views in a calmer setting. George really welcomed my follow-up visit.

"Mr. Munro, my wife and I are from Indiana and we have had problems adjusting to Alaska and also working at this hospital."

"Coming recently from California, I can relate to what you're saying. However, in terms of work, or personal issues, what is your most pressing problem?"

"May I speak openly and honestly with you? I am very upset and confused."

"Yes, you have my loyalty and confidentiality!"

Sadly and almost tearfully, he said, "I feel so inferior."

"You are a nice-looking young man, you have good manners, and you present yourself well. You also appear self-assured. What is the problem?"

"My brother. I am definitely certain that he is my parent's favorite son. In school he was one of the most outstanding athletes—good at everything. Everything seemed centered around him. We attended all of his sporting events, with my parents—particularly my father—constantly bragging and raving about how wonderful he was. No one said anything good about me. I was like standing in the corner—a nobody."

"Where and what is your brother, today?"

"He is a drug addict and in a rehabilitation unit in Florida."

"This is my plan for you. We have an employee referral service that you can use at no cost. I want to arrange a treatment plan for you where you can discuss your problems and get some expert counseling. Are you willing to work with me in initiating this program?"

"Yes!"

"I'll continue to support you through this process. However, my observation, simply being a layperson, is the following: I strongly believe your parents, in earlier years, sagaciously and confidentially identified some weak areas in your brother's personality. Therefore, they determined the need to support him in every way—including the need to strongly recognize his success as an athlete. They were probably trying, very discreetly, to give him recognition, to try and booster his fragile self-esteem."

In his reaction to these comments, he looked to me as if he were thinking: *Mr. Munro—a nice thoughtful man, but bonkers in his assessment.*

However, more importantly, he proceeded with the treatment plan, overlooking my frivolous assessment.

George and his wife shortly thereafter had a baby. George's parents came for a visit to see their new grandchild. The following day, George came rushing into my office beaming euphorically. "Mr. Munro, my father pulled me aside last night to talk to me privately. He told me that he and my mother were so proud of me. My father said that it had always been imperative that they devote more time to my brother so they could support his shaky ego. He realized that they'd overlooked my needs for reassurance, but they knew I 'had it all together.' My father said exactly what you told me. I couldn't believe it, and I couldn't wait to get to work this morning to tell you. Your observations were right on target."

"I am so happy for you. I believe being an observer simply comes more easily as one is removed from the pain and suffering. Enjoy your visit with your parents."

Because of the new baby, George was encouraged by his family to return to Indiana. He called me from Indiana and said something to the effect that he wanted to return to Anchorage some day because he had Mr. Munro for support and guidance. I told him that I would call him if any open positions became available. My comments were mendacious, as I knew that he was just experiencing "resettlement pains." I never ever heard from him again. He was a nice lad, and I enjoyed working with him.

While in Alaska, I was notified that my mother had expired. Unknown to me, she had been ill for several months and, I believe, had been hospitalized in an extended-care facility. Upon receiving notification of her demise, I was also informed that there would be no funeral service to attend. Before I moved to Alaska, the same year as my move, my niece Robin and I had been in Vancouver attending the World's Fair. We had made arrangements to meet with my mother for dinner one evening during our brief stay in that city and we had had a nice visit.

I had moved on from that devastating time when I was three and arrived home from the hospital to find I suddenly was part of a single-parent family. There was little to remember prior to that time. But neither had there been any feeling of reconciliation.

Shortly after my grandmother passed away, my sister Marjorie was to receive a small set of china that my father had given my grandmother. Marjorie informed my mother that she really had no need for it. My mother called me and asked if I would like it as a keepsake in memory of my grandmother. My very first acrimonious response, after years of superficial bullshit, was,

"Perhaps I would prefer from you some appropriate recognition for all of the years that I had to spend doing duties you normally should have fulfilled."

Taken back, she had caustically responded, "I will have to think about that comment."

I equally sardonically replied, "If that is the case, I suggest you forget about it."

Again, there was never any conciliatory bonding between my mother and me. We had a very shallow relationship. We spent time together socially; she was my mother, but in name only. Her contribution to my wellbeing had ended the day that cheater arrived in our bedroom all those years ago. I believe we get what we give! And she received nothing from me. Prior to starting my visits to her home, she apparently had seen Marjorie and me on the street while driving past us. Her comment was, "We were on our way somewhere and didn't have time to stop." Hearing those impersonal blasé comments, I realized we were no "big deal" to her.

In looking back, my sister Laura was blessed with my mother's beautiful dark brown eyes and flawlessly white skin. Both women had excellent taste in dress and always looked immaculately and outstandingly well groomed. Their good looks dated back to my very handsome grandfather. In terms of complimentary comments to my mother, I always said she was the second best housekeeper in Canada, her mother being my number-one favorite. My mother had perfect table manners. My sister Marjorie, in appearance, is a Munro, although she shared my mother and Laura's good grooming qualities. Years ago while still in Canada, I met a man from her office and asked if he knew my sister, Marjorie Munro.

He responded, "Daily I come to work, look at her, and think I should go home and shower. She is so immaculately groomed!" (Not bad considering she'd been "half-assed" raised by Dad and me.)

In terms of my mother, I believe that she was in denial regarding what we three children faced subsequent to the events that followed my father's return home that horrible night. She remarried and she presumably had a wonderful and fulfilling happy life. Her solace was directing anger at my father.

Her leaving my father was never the issue with me. The issue was the circumstances in which those events occurred. We were young children and everyone was involved in the midst of a horrible Depression. In terms of the aftermath, I was happy to be able to stick with my dad.

My sister Marjorie has been a wonderful mother, as are both of her daughters, Robin and Michele. I truly never ever wanted a family. Finally, after twenty-three years, I was free for the first time in my life.

Every year, each Alaskan who had been in the state for a twelve-month period was entitled to an oil revenue dividend check. Each person would have another person sign a form attesting that that person had been in the state for twelve months. While I was in Alaska, the check was about one thousand dollars, so a family of two adults and three children would receive five thousand dollars—a great gift.

Some check-cashing local organizations would provide a service to those persons who needed funds badly by advancing them the amount of their dividend check, deducting their fee in the process. I assume they calculated their fee based on the length of time they had to wait for the check to arrive, which was in October. That type of service offered by cash and loan companies had a negative impact on the community generally at that time.

We offered a special program for people who wished to settle their indebtedness to the hospital when the oil revenue dividend checks were due. In some cases, we would match their funds in discharging their bills. The local TV news station sent their interviewers and camera crew to our hospital. Our administration always freely volunteered my services. I was elected to discuss the program on camera.

Fortunately, I wore a suit every day because I never knew what was going to happen from one day to the next. Everything in Anchorage seemed to be addressed spontaneously and sometimes erratically, or it could be that we were heavily involved with the media, as we resided in Alaska's largest community.

One morning I was asked to come to the administration department immediately to meet with one of our media persons. She informed me that one of our local newspaper writers would be coming to interview me in a few minutes regarding the Medicaid program in the State of Alaska. This newspaper representative, although I didn't know it at the time, was a prominent writer, and her husband was a renowned local radio newscaster.

I was led to believe that this lady could be very difficult, and I muttered, "Thanks for the very short notice."

She arrived and we quickly had a lengthy session, and everything went great. At the end of the meeting, I walked her to her car. (I always felt accompanying visitors to their cars exemplified a personal touch.) She asked me a couple of additional questions, which I answered.

She came on two other occasions. Her articles were voluminously written with my name and quotations prominently and favorably and very accurately mentioned. She turned out to be one of the nicest persons. She often called me for my remarks, both off and on the record. She was a sweetheart and a very bright and articulate lady. She knew her craft and performed beautifully and ethically. She was anything but difficult. It was always a joy to meet interesting people such as this lady from the media.

One day our administrative media people asked that I join them that evening to appear on a talk radio program. I was unfamiliar with the program and the host. During the day, my colleagues informed me that the radio host was very difficult, opinionated, and obnoxious. We arrived together at the radio station. I soon learned that the broadcast premises were under tight security, and all entrances were locked at all times. We were taken to a refreshment bar area and someone pointed out our radio host to me as he passed by with a frown on his face.

The program started and, after about ten minutes, the host started to warm up to us. He informed his radio audience that he was looking at three very sincere individuals. He was gregarious and charming throughout the rest of the program. One of my employees called in to specifically ask questions regarding a state program, which afforded me the opportunity to express my views. She did this spontaneously, and I was grateful to her for her insight and for taking the initiative to call the program.

When I first arrived in Alaska, I was totally confused regarding Medicaid and their General Relief programs. I arranged to meet a couple of specialists for lunch a few weeks after starting at the hospital. I had heard a lot of gobbledygook about the programs and I am a just-give-me-the-facts-only-and-skip-the-rest person. At lunch with the specialists and one of my managers, I asked that we start backwards on both programs—I will tell you about our programs in California and you tell me how they relate to yours. Using my approach, I put it all together over lunch and repeated to them their programs, addressing all of the salient points.

Aside from bringing my areas of responsibility to an acceptable level, I was also asked to conduct a class for newcomers to nursing services. I conducted the class once a month and I enjoyed being involved; however, it wasn't adroitly planned on my part in terms of priority. I would receive last-minute reminders that it was nearly time for class. I never planned the presentation. Aside from being constantly overwhelmed with so many projects, the students by late afternoon had heavy eyelids and were ready for a lulling presentation.

For some strange reason, as soon as I appeared before the class, I became animated and randomly selected a topic of interest. I covered managed care, Medicare and Medicaid, and the Alaskan General Relief program, and a lot of historical information covering healthcare over my many years of experience.

Quite suddenly the heavy eyelids would open; my presentations were very well received. Strangely enough, this situation seemed to happen at each class, and was somewhat surprising to me. It afforded me the impetus to really put my best foot forward, so to speak.

Throughout one session, a very inquiring nurse kept firing questions at me and I couldn't discern if she found my material engrossing or if she was challenging my presentation and comments. The dialogue between us kept coming because of her prerogative. I was somewhat bewildered as to my effectiveness during this ongoing exchange.

At the end of the class, up went her hand once more. She asked, "Have you ever taught classes at the university?"

I replied, "No!"

She said, "I want you to know that I have learned more in this class today than I have in all of the other classes that I have attended at the university covering the same or similar subject material. I cannot tell you how much I have enjoyed being in your class today. I am grateful that you also fully answered my questions. I sincerely hope you teach at the university—they really need you."

Needless to say, I was quite surprised and pleased with her flattering remarks. I did have one opportunity to teach a class at the university as their guest speaker for the hour. Nursing administration informed hospital administration that I was considered one of the most popular teachers in their program—based on student comments. Oddly enough, during my years in Alaska my lackadaisical approach in teaching the class consistently won me four stars. It was not bad testimony for this grade-school dropout to receive.

Actually, and sometime later in California, a local college was very interested in my conducting classes for their students, solely based on my reputation through my hospital. Their commendation in trying to recruit me was appreciated; however, I had other commitments to address that would have been too conflicting. But it lingered in the back of my mind for some time.

As I had in California, in Alaska I conducted meetings in the community covering our services and Medicare and other payers. These meetings took place during the week in the late afternoon or early evening. When they occurred, they were simply an extension of my working day. However, I was asked to make a presentation at one of the military bases in Anchorage on a Saturday morning. The meeting was to address the Champus program and other healthcare plans. Because it was a Saturday morning, I viewed it as an informal gathering and I wore Nordstrom's tasteful but casual dress. I wore a long-sleeve shirt that I buttoned up, but I didn't wear a tie or jacket.

When I arrived compulsively early, I noticed that all of the men were in either uniform or suits (spit and polish, so to speak) and the ladies were commensurately well dressed. I thought to myself, *Oh, my God!* Appearance and decorum are so important to me, and I was a director representing the largest hospital in Alaska. And I realized that military personnel have rigid standards.

We were awaiting three other speakers from the community. Prior to their arrival, I took the opportunity to mingle with the audience. They were very gracious and friendly and I realized that most of my discomfort was probably self-imposed; however, I was surprised but frankly elated when the other speakers arrived. They were too old to be called ragamuffins, but their casual dress was nondescript—old slacks and sweaters that made them look as if they were heading for the bush country. Talk about a motley crew! They made and saved my day. My God, they looked dreadful. I was so happy and grateful to them; by contrast, I looked terrific.

When I first started at Providence Hospital in Anchorage, I received a letter from a very disgruntled employee who apparently had been moved repeatedly hither and yon within the organization. When I started to read her letter, I thought it had been typed and prepared by an eight-year-old who was trying to learn how to type and spell simultaneously. It was unequivocally the worst written message I have ever attempted to read. It was unbelievable; some parts were actually undecipherable. I did not get to meet with this lady, as she decided to seek employment elsewhere. I believe her letter was sent to me in both anger and frustration, and as a last-ditch stand; however, it was so ineptly written that it lost its purpose.

Apparently, she was applying for a position at a medical group on the outskirts of the city. I had just read the letter when I received a call from one of the physicians in the group asking for a reference. I informed him that I was new to the hospital and that his applicant had not worked under my supervision.

I also informed him that any requests for references should be directed through our human resources department. From the tone of his voice I detected a somewhat confrontational attitude; I tended to believe that he had tried other sources and frustratingly had not come up with any help in measuring this applicant's worthiness.

He said he was interested in the applicant, as she had been with the hospital for several years. He wondered why she would have remained there all that time if her work was unsatisfactory. Thought I silently, *Undisputedly, a very good question.* I was tempted to suggest to him that she send him a letter stating why she would like to work in his medical group. Unfortunately, I could only refer him back to our human resources department simply for a verification of employment. Discreetness takes precedence in these touchy situations.

There was a wonderful director in charge of our human resources department when I first arrived at Anchorage, and she was a great help to me. The hospital had accommodated my move to Alaska and there were a few minor problems relating to the transportation of my furnishings. Marty immediately contacted the local representative at the transfer service and got everything straightened out.

The spring and summer days are very long in Alaska, compared to the very short days in fall and winter. I went walking virtually every night all year. One spring evening as I was walking, I suddenly ran into Marty, who was doing the same thing. We both were speed walkers. After the first walk, she suggested that we walk together on a regular basis.

Marty was very petite and, in appearance, strongly resembled Judy Garland. She had been in Anchorage for several years and had recently and unhappily ended a ten-year marriage. As I was much older, our relationship was purely platonic. During the week, after work, in the warmer months, we would speed walk and hike in the wooded hills near our condos. On weekends, we would head for the mountains or other recreational areas when I finished work in the early or late afternoon. She really knew the outdoors in the surrounding Anchorage area. We had great fun and our treks were always a new experience for me. We would run into moose on the trails while enjoying the wild flowers, foliage, and berries. We would pause to admire the wonderful expansive scenery of deciduous bushes and trees.

When we completed our weekend hiking, I would suggest we go for Mexican food with margaritas or to other restaurants that we had learned to favor. As neither of us had a weight problem, I loved to devour what I could, and she would join me to a lesser degree. After each weekend dinner, she would look at me and say, "You have ruined our day with your gluttony and we must now go walking for at least another hour or so." I liked her no-BS comments and attitude—straight to the point. I loved her femininity and enjoyed teasing her. I can assure you, after our feasts we walked much more slowly—speed walking was *verboten*.

Unfortunately for me, Marty moved back to her home state of New York while I was still in Alaska. She was so special and I really missed her. She was great fun and we did speed walk one year in the Anchorage Marathon. We did very well, arriving in the walker's vanguard—she in her thirties and I in my fifties.

When I worked in Oxnard and resided in Ventura, I could find excellent Mexican food and restaurants on every other corner. Many of my employees were of Hispanic background and truly knew how to prepare their family dishes. Everyone teased me at SJRMC when I announced my plans to move to Alaska. They were sure that I would miss my margaritas and Mexican food. At first I did, but then I seemed to get used to the Mexican restaurants in Alaska. When in Rome! If I decided to leave Alaska, my parting words would be, "I have to return to California because the Mexican food is starting to taste good in Alaska; I must have developed a very serious gourmet problem."

Needless to say, having four tennis courts at my disposal, I had spent a lot of time on the courts in Ventura. In Anchorage, I had tennis colleagues at work, and I played with one of the professors at the University of Alaska. I was definitely a baseline player and rallied well and constantly. I was much in demand during the long daylight months. However, I got so acclimated to the scenery and wild life in Anchorage that I would decline tennis invitations to go hiking through the backwoods. My professor friend and other tennis colleagues at work were not too happy.

I had had another professor tennis friend in Ventura. He was an amazing powerhouse in whacking that ball over the net and he was a rallying dynamo. Ironically, that energetic individual was an ornithologist—a profession whose members are occasionally stereotyped as intellectually meek individuals with thick rimmed glasses, a bird book in one hand, and field glasses in the other, but not as a robust tennis player. He said I matched his brawn!

One Saturday, after leaving my Providence Hospital office, I stopped by the tennis courts to hit on the backboard. While I was working out, a nice lady approached me and asked if I had another tennis racket with me. Before I could respond, she said, "I am visiting here from Westchester County in New York and I play tennis regularly." We just rallied for about an hour or so and chatted intermittently. I mentioned to her that I was with the hospital and she informed me that she was visiting with one of our physicians and his family, and mentioned his name. I said that I knew him professionally at the hospital and that he was also one of my personal physicians.

She mentioned that her lifelong ambition had been to purchase land in Alaska on a river for a summer retreat. She had just completed that goal and was training the doctor's children and some of their friends to ice skate. We agreed to meet the following day at the tennis courts and, after tennis, we would go hiking in my favorite backcountry.

In meeting new people I am somewhat reserved and not too curious by nature regarding their backgrounds. I could tell that this lady was definitely "outdoorsy." I was right; when we went for our hike the following day, she was in her element. We hiked through the hills and I showed her the small gushing falls and the narrow rivers where the salmon come to spawn. I also showed her a place on the river where you can cross on a fallen log—explaining that the salmon sometimes get deterred when they try to get under the log to continue their voyage upstream. I also mentioned that I had met another hiker who had been on the (American Olympic) skiing team and he had taken me hiking originally in that area. She was enjoying the tour and the wilderness immensely, which was gratifying to me.

I said, "Aside from fulfilling your Alaskan dreams, who are you and what do you do in Westchester County, New York?"

"I'm a speed skating instructor."

"Do you work with hockey teams and individuals?"

She said, "Yes!"

I jokingly said, "Have you ever worked with Wayne Gretzky?"

Again, she said, "Yes!" She informed me that she traveled extensively throughout the United States and Canada. She had even worked with a hockey team my cousins had played on—Manitoba's finest, the Flin Flon Bombers. When I returned to California for Christmas vacation, I mentioned her to one of my Canadian friends who was a former boxer and an ardent hockey (et al.) sports fan. He informed me that she was well known in the sports world as an outstanding and prestigious speed skating coach.

It is important to develop good relationships with our insurance intermediaries. The two hospitals I had been involved with in Southern California had shared the same intermediaries, and the relationships that I had developed with them over the years remained in tact when I moved from one hospital to the other. The outpost to Alaska is Seattle. Blue Cross is located there and they were the intermediaries for Medicare and the Champus programs along with their various Blue Cross plans.

We worked closely with the governmental agencies administrative people in Juneau regarding the Medicaid and General Relief programs. Fortunately the claims processing was done in Anchorage, and at a location fairly close to the hospital.

I made periodic visits to Seattle to meet with the Blue Cross representatives regarding their programs and claims processing. Those visits were instrumental in further establishing an excellent working relationship with those involved.

I also traveled to Juneau to discuss important issues relating to programs for the indigent, with governmental persons responsible for them. I routinely followed the claims processing locally. It rains incessantly in Juneau, but the city has the quaintness of Carmel with several small pastry and coffee shops. It is very picturesque, but remotely located. I enjoyed working with members of our state government in Juneau. Unlike the representatives in California, they were very accessible because Alaska is a less-populated state and our hospital was vitally important to Alaskans.

Before moving to Alaska, I had traveled several times by plane, but I still had a terrible fear of flying. Through one of my social services colleagues at SJRMC, I was put in touch with a program conducted at LAX for people who suffered with a fear of flying. It was about a four-hour session, which was held at a large hotel near LAX. The instructor was a commercial pilot and also a psychologist.

The course was well attended and, after about a two-hour session, we went to LAX and boarded a plane. We sat on the stationary plane for about an hour and returned back to the hotel classroom for the remainder of the session.

It was helpful to me, as I traveled extensively from Alaska to the lower forty-eight states during my years in Anchorage. The trip I most feared was to Juneau, as the plane cuts short when landing and taking off between the thin coastline and the mountain range. Fortunately, I was pre-warned by a colleague at the hospital, who also had a fear of flying, regarding arriving and departing Juneau.

When my friend Marty left Alaska, I inherited her Alaska Airlines mileage upgrades. In most cases, I was able to use those credits for first-class service, also simultaneously building more mileage credits. Fortunately, because of her gift, I traveled in the first-class section where the drinks flowed freely. As I was met at each end and with no driving involved, I was usually higher than the plane. The liquor helped reduce my great anguish in my fear of flying.

At Providence Hospital we had a large neonatal intensive care unit, which was extensively used throughout the year. Many infants were either born in our hospital or flown in from all parts of the state. The parents of many of these infants resided in remote villages. For the parents who came to Anchorage, the journey was equivalent to someone from the sticks arriving in New York City. It was really overwhelming to the native population having to come to Anchorage and having to apply for medical assistance.

The State of Alaska did provide free medical services to the Native American Indian and Eskimo population through the native hospital and medical facilitates. They also provided services on transferred patients from the native hospital to our private facility; however, the infant care cases were paid through Medicaid and we had to directly work with the families and/or their representatives.

I was very fortunate to have a patient representative from the native hospital assigned at our facility to assist us in working with the Native American Indian and Eskimo population. This native lady was extremely bright, and she spoke several dialects and communicated beautifully with our native patients and/or their representatives.

This very talented lady had one shortcoming—she had a tendency to imbibe. It was everyone's desire to keep her on the straight and narrow path as her communicative services were so desperately needed by a special segment of the population. Having been transferred from the Native Hospital (but still remaining their employee) she knew all of the staff at that facility. She was a great facilitator at each end, having worked in both hospitals.

Sadly, she came to visit me one morning to tell me that she had been discharged from her position. She arrived late to work. When she routinely reported to the other facility, she mentioned that she had imbibed after hours and that was the reason for her tardiness. Evidently, this had been one of many issues, and I desperately tried to get her reinstated, as she was so valuable to our facility. I was distraught for days at the loss of this talented linguistic native lady. Being resourceful, she devoted her time to making native arts and crafts from her home. She occasionally stopped by to see me and, on one occasion, separated me from millions of other men when she departed from my office—she showed her affection for me by rubbing noses with me. It was a very unique and complimentary experience for this Anglo-Saxon. Losing this talented linguist was, sadly, an immeasurable loss.

Native crafts are very expensive and, over the years, have greatly appreciated in value. While living in Alaska I purchased some crafts from native Alaskans who surreptitiously would wander through the hospital with some of their items and discreetly approach certain individuals. This was totally frowned upon by our administration, but I broke the rules a few times in obtaining some great gift items. I tried to apply common sense when viewing these situations.

I could readily identify the native freelance artisans and I would rush them into my office to examine their merchandise. A "squealer" once reported that I had a "skulker" in my office. I wormed my way out of it by saying that it was important to support native artisans, who were working independently to support their craft. It worked—I think? There were only a few artisans involved, and their visits were rare.

Also, the Native Hospital Gift Shop that I strongly supported sold arts and crafts much less expensively than commercial stores and gift shops did. In terms of native crafts, my experience was related to Alaska only. Actually, I have made it a habit over the years to shop at quality hospital gift shops to purchase items. Most of their staffing does represent volunteers, thus, the overhead for payroll is lower and quality items are generally more reasonably priced.

20

Each year, my gift to my employees in Alaska was a special luncheon prior to Christmas. Upon my arrival to the hospital, Richard had a new business office under construction along with admitting services in a very centralized area in the main building. When we relocated to our new facility, a large kitchen area and extended counter space and shelving had been added to the project. The kitchen and counter space were actually centrally located among three departmental units, which was very conducive for buffet luncheons.

I selected two fastidious ladies to join me in arranging the Christmas luncheon. I took them both to outside markets where we ordered special trays of veggies and cold cuts, fruit, and snack trays, desserts, and nonalcoholic beverages. We purchased plastic dinnerware, cups, napkins, and other table items internally. The two ladies listened carefully to me regarding the logistics of picking up our orders from the markets and arranging the departmental setup and completing the food preparation and making the punch and so on.

The first year, as I had over seventy employees, I had a meeting a few days prior to the luncheon. I informed my folks that they could invite other persons to the luncheon as their guests; however, they should let us know if they invited a guest so that we had plenty of food and beverages. I personally invited several key persons myself. It was very successful and everyone really enjoyed this new event.

The following year, the two ladies, when we arrived at the market, informed me that I could wheel the cart and open my wallet, but that would be the full extent of my participation. At preparation time they gave me the bum's rush and informed me that I was simply the host of the luncheon. On the day of the event I asked if I could make the punch or do anything to help. They told me to just leave and do my job as host.

The number of guests increased about twofold the second year. I had informed both ladies from the start the prior year, that I did not want the embarrassment of running out of food or drink. They were great in their anticipation regarding the ordering of necessary additional amounts. Those ladies were wonderful and I can only take credit for selecting them as they did a superb job.

The Christmas luncheon became one of the most popular events of the season throughout the hospital. It created a tremendous amount of much needed goodwill for my departments. After the event, I always flew to California for Christmas.

The husband of Susie, one of the luncheon ladies, worked in his brother-in-law's service station, which also was equipped with a carwash and provided detailing services. They were a nice family, all originally for Georgia. Because of the inclement weather in Alaska and the awful amount of dirt and grime produced during the April thawing breakup, my leased car was ready every spring for a complete detailing job.

The first time I took my vehicle to this family carwash, Susie notified them in advance of my visit, informing them that my automobile needed to be shining both inside and out when it was returned to me. When I arrived, everyone said, "Susie called us." One of them laughed and said, "We have been fully instructed."

They were so meticulous, they were still doing a last-minute rub just as I was driving off. I had never ever received such VIP treatment. I was impressed and somewhat embarrassed. I had that automobile for almost four years. When I turned it in, the leasing agent said it looked brand new. It was all due to low mileage and my annual detailing.

When you befriend Alaskans—whether they're Alaskans by birth or transplant—they stick by you. People were wonderful to me in Alaska and I appreciated their kindness and sincerity.

While I was at SJRMC, my great friend Linda was Richard's secretary. When I was in Alaska, a lady named Lydia was secretary to Richard, and she and I became immediate friends. She was divorced and originated from Munich, but, after many years in Alaska, her English was flawless. Also, like Linda, she had a great sense of humor and we had a lot of fun together.

One evening we went for dinner. I was the first to arrive. I removed my storm coat and placed it on the restaurant coat rack and waited for her at our table. After dinner, she realized that I had left my coat in the foyer. As I was putting it on she informed me in a lecturing manner never to leave my coat again. I was always to take it to the booth with me because someone might take it. She was still lecturing as we drove off and I didn't pay too much attention to her.

The following evening before leaving the office, I stopped by my assistant director's office to say good night and to have some last minute conversation. Suddenly, I put my hand in my storm coat and pulled out a set of keys. I said, "Where did these come from?"

My assistant immediately said, "Where did you have dinner last night?"

I felt so stupid as I suddenly realized I had taken someone else's coat from the rack.

I called the restaurant and was informed that the other guest had taken my coat. He'd left his name and hotel, as he was a visiting hockey coach from the lower forty-eight. When I delivered his coat, he laughed when I informed him that I had been cautioned about keeping my own coat from being stolen, when in fact, I had, at the same time, been stealing his. Lydia shook her head but laughed when I told her of my blunder. That restaurant served the best Italian food I have ever eaten—and in Alaska yet!

One evening Lydia and I were invited to her married daughter's home. She whispered to me that they were all very young people, and if other mature adults did not arrive, we would be leaving early. The young folks were in their twenties and were great fun. I ended up on the floor with them laughing, teasing, and telling stories. We quickly developed a great rapport. My friend realized I was having fun and we stayed, but she glared at me most of the evening to let me know she was more than ready to leave.

There was a large community of Germans living in Anchorage. One evening, Lydia and I had been invited to dinner at one of their homes. They were nice, but complete strangers, and I felt shy and withdrawn. Presumably to get even with me for our prolonged stay at her daughter's party, after dinner Lydia shockingly announced that I would sing "Lili Marleen." I sang the German version in English and Lydia said later (failing to mention that her plot had backfired) that I had been the hit of the evening. One man, who had been in the German army, found it reminiscent and he and the other guests loved it. Lydia loved challenging me. We always shared great humorous social times together.

When I first started working in Alaska, I reported to an interim person. That person and I did not develop an unequivocally good rapport. My areas of responsibility upon arrival were a chaotic mess. While I will not dwell on those circumstances, I will say that I found that the person to whom I temporarily reported had a very condescending attitude toward me. My perception was that 95 percent of this attitude was a defense mechanism, as in her regular areas of responsibility she was proficient and highly respected. My areas of responsibility were virtually unfamiliar to her.

One late afternoon shortly after I started, she requested that I write a revised detailed specific standard practice procedure. She said it was imperative that I have it on her desk by early morning. I worked late into the evening, but had it completed by morning. I met her in her office. She did not say good morning or show any other amenities; she just took the document, did a cursory review, accepted it, and said nothing.

My candid and observant friend Lydia had sensed that I displayed an air of phoniness in trying to ingratiate myself with this person. She was absolutely right. A similar incident occurred, and it became the icing on the cake. In plain English, I informed the interim person where she could stuff my job. Apparently, she panicked during our obstreperous one-way conversation, realizing that I was not going to take any "BS" from her. She ran in panic to Richard and asked him to intercede.

The following day, Richard stopped by my office and said that his family wanted me to join them for dinner at the ice rink. He suggested that after dinner we adults would go elsewhere for dessert and coffee.

When Richard, his wife, and I settled alone I said, "I know why we are here."

He resoundingly said, "What can I do to help you to mitigate this situation?"

"Nothing. I am, facetiously speaking, trying to turn this lady into a goddess and it isn't going to happen overnight."

It all worked out, as we were both good at our respective positions but both Scorpios with clashing personalities. We Scorpios seem to either connect or disconnect. For some reason, we never allow for a middle ground.

Lydia had the final word after that truculent confrontation, "What happened? She's so cheerful in the mornings and says good morning to everyone now every day." I surmised that, to counter my unflattering comments, she had decided to present herself in a more favorable light. Great!

Upon my arrival to Anchorage and, of course, at the hospital, Richard and his wife and family sort of adopted me. I became Uncle Gus. I had had a lifelong habit of placing all of my coinage each day in a kitchen tin. I never kept coinage in my pocket to spend. When I lived in California, when the tin was nearly full, I would take it to my nieces for spending money. In Alaska, I gave my coinage to Richard's children. The first time I gave it to them, the children were together sitting on the floor and I simply dumped the coins out onto the carpet.

One said, "I'll count the quarters and pennies; you count the dimes, and nickels."

When they finished counting, one of them shouted, "We have over $140 and change!"

They loved it and looked forward to my "tin can visits."

On one occasion, Richard's oldest daughter Kim asked to speak with me privately. She wondered if I could assist her in getting a job at the hospital when she completed her high school classes at the end of the term. She had had a part-time job the previous summer and had actually been sent to one of my departments to help on a special project. I suggested she come and meet with me in my office near the end of the term and we would work it out. Richard knew nothing of this plan until the time arrived; then Kim discussed it with him.

Richard called me one morning after learning of this proposed plan. "Gus, Kim tells me that you are hiring her for the summer months to work in one of your departments."

"Yes, that's correct."

"Gus, I don't believe that it would be prudent for her to accept that position."

"Why?"

"Kim worked last year and there were some concerns in certain quarters."

"Richard, I assume from your vagueness you are referring to nepotism?"

"Yes!"

"Dick, trust me. I do not play games. Kim has excellent skills and I am not going to deprive her of this opportunity just because she just happens to be your daughter. I report to you; Kim will report to me."

"Gus, I feel uncomfortable." And he added a few more vague comments.

"Richard, Kim needs a summer job and I need her services—it is that simple. I also take full responsibility and you can refer anyone who has a concern to me."

"Gus, this situation concerns me; however, I shall leave it in your court."

Quoting the legendary actor, Humphrey Bogart, "Tennis anyone?"

Kim spent the summer with us. She did a great job and my folks loved her. Her proud father would occasionally stop by and inquire about Kim's performance or he would stop by simply just to drive her home. I think I had learned my lesson about this situation from Martha at SJRMC, when she went over my head and hired my niece Robin. In both cases everything worked out very well.

During the school year, Kim was studying psychological testing. Richard had been one of her guinea pigs and, when I arrived at their home for dinner one evening, he suggested to Kim that she give me the same test she had just given him. Kim banished her father from the room and we got down to work. As soon as I finished answering her multiple-choice questions, Richard reentered the room and was eager to see my scoring.

"I knew it!" said he, when Kim gave him the results. "Gus, you and I have scored almost identically with each other. We think so much alike!"

"Both Scorpios too!"

This was very complimentary to me, as he was an articulate and decent man. I believe he liked my tenaciousness and my no-BS attitude—though he would have worded that differently. Dick was a very religious man and blissfully practiced his faith daily.

A young man named Robert was the assistant manager in admitting when I arrived in Alaska. He and his wife had met in Anchorage when they were both in the air force. Upon discharge from the service, he started his civilian career at Providence Hospital.

They had three small children and were homeschooling their oldest child. Robert was in his late twenties and I sensed that he had a tremendous potential. Unfortunately, as the assistant manager, and being in a subordinate position, he was in an awkward position, having to placate the person to whom he reported.

As time passed, changes occurred and Robert reported to an interim person. One late afternoon, I met with him and the interim admitting manager, along with my assistant director. I sort of read them the riot act in terms of addressing the needs of the admitting personnel. It was nothing to do with Robert, but a quarrelsome situation had arisen between the department head and the staff. When the meeting ended, I suggested that we four go for dinner at our favorite Mexican restaurant.

Late the following afternoon, my patient representative supervisor stopped by and said she had just spoken with Robert, who was upset. Robert told her that he didn't understand me. He told her that we had had a very heated meeting in which I had laid down the law, and then I had taken everyone to dinner. He stated that, at the restaurant, I was laughing and having a good time as if nothing had happened. He said to her, "I don't understand Gus! What are your thoughts on him?"

She had responded, "Yes, he has definite views on work-related issues, but he can separate work from fun and have a pleasant evening. He is opinionated, but very fair and usually right."

Sometime later, Robert and his wife decided to return to New Jersey. He stopped by to tell me his plans. Realizing his potentiality, I called a colleague in Los Angeles, who had contacts in New Jersey. Together we located a hospital that had a possible position for him.

Before leaving Alaska, Robert waited until he received the state dividend checks that amounted to about five thousand dollars for his family. They left Alaska in November and drove partway to board a ship that would take them to a port in British Columbia. When they began the driving trip from Anchorage to the port, it was snowing and the landscape was completely desolate and bleak. His youngest son looked around and inquired, "Dad, are you sure this is the right road to New Jersey?" His parents laughed heartily, as his comments were justifiably profound. My parting gift was a two-day stay in Vancouver at the Sylvia Hotel, a designated heritage site. They stayed in one of the small family apartments and loved it. (I also stayed there as a guest on trips to Vancouver and always looked forward to those stays.)

As children, Cecil and I always had admired that ivy-covered hotel at English Bay. We passed it en route to Second Beach to swim in their ocean water pool.

In the workplace, I had always been sort of a control freak in terms of getting things done and not relying on other individuals. My team of supervisors and I at SJRMC, had had one goal, and that was to get the job done with no excuses. We all pitched in and worked together to keep on track and to be up to date throughout the office. In working with my assistant in Alaska, I heard a lot of platitudes in the wake of the computer conversion. People kept saying that it takes time to bring everything up to date after such a change. I started to identify these comments in terms of the blasé attitude displayed by one or two of our supervisors, and this disturbed me.

My assistant wanted more responsibility in order to gain more experience in the day-to-day operations, and I slackened the reins to let her get more involved. My tenure in remaining in Alaska was precarious and I was happy to elevate her position to replace me, if I were to decide to return to the lower forty-eight.

She started working with a new supervisor, who was from a medical office. In a short period of time, the new supervisor and I had developed a good rapport. I found her to be an excellent person: dedicated, knowledgeable, and extremely affable. Unfortunately, she and my assistant clashed, and the new supervisor informed me that she could not work with her. She stated that she totally concurred with whatever I requested on how to achieve our goals. I tried to encourage her to continue working with my assistant to see if they could develop a better working relationship. I liked them both, and I optimistically believed that, with some effort, they could march in tandem together.

That was not the case. The supervisor turned in her resignation and, unbeknownst to me, requested a meeting with the director of human resources and our CFO together to discuss her reasons for her resignation. She informed them that I was outstanding and great to work with, and she then discussed my assistant in negative terms. I believe the CFO had approved my expansion of my assistant's role, but had some reservations. Unfortunately, this adroit lady made a very compelling case that placed my assistant in a somewhat untenable position. Apparently, she was only one of a vanguard of discontented people to vocalize frustration. Shortly thereafter, my assistant resigned and left Alaska, and I was faced with looking for a new assistant. Unfortunately, I lost the new supervisor too.

There was a very bright and proficient lady, Charlotte, who administered a professional billing unit for physicians. She was also responsible for the specialized billing for our air services, and she had very close ties with our accounting department. From time to time, my folks would need to contact her on certain issues. They invariably complained of her obstreperous demeanor when they approached her on issues relating to her areas of responsibility. At the time, I did not know her, but my gut feeling was that she was a diamond in the rough and really knew her work. When confronted with complaints regarding her seemingly caustic mannerisms and/or lack of affability, I would always ask, "Did she help you?"

And the answer was always, "Yes!"

Any conversations I had had with Charlotte had been pleasant and straightforward. I met with her and informed her that I would be interested in having her join our department as my assistant. I further stated that I believe she had the proper qualifications.

Her reply was, "They hate me!"

I said, "Forget all of that—please come and work with us." And she did.

I must add that even routine recruitment in Anchorage was difficult, and Charlotte was a golden find to me.

Our first encounter occurred just shortly after she accepted her new position. She and I had been meeting with one of her doctors regarding some professional billing issues. The doctor asked me a question and I responded, "I don't know the answer, but I will check it out and get back to you."

After the meeting she said, "I can't believe you told him that you didn't know the answer."

I replied, "What's so strange about that?"

Charlotte was totally bewildered at my honesty, thinking I should have come up with some kind of an answer. Needless to say, she and I had a long discussion on the subject. I said, "You build respect with everyone by being truthful and, most importantly, by following through with information—in a timely fashion."

Charlotte was scheduled to make a presentation to Richard and some of his administrative colleagues on some professional billing issues. She had become noticeably more comfortable with me and had virtually dropped her guard. Just before her presentation, she stopped by my office insisting that I come to the meeting with her. I asked in a routine manner why she needed me, as she knew all of the answers and I had nothing further to contribute. "I need your moral support when I am confronted with the administrative staff. I don't feel comfortable alone with them."

At meeting time, I smiled and mockingly said, "You don't need me—but let's go."

From that day forth, I became her best friend at the hospital. She was a very bright and talented lady and was loaded with integrity—and nervous energy, like me!

One morning, as I arrived to work—via her department—she pointed to one of our computers. I said, "It looks like you are running off your bills instead of data processing?"

"You got that right—I can't be messing around with them this morning—I need bills immediately." Our morning encounters predictably included her litany of woes.

Charlotte was incredible, but a brazen brat; however, I adored her. Also, she was consistently both forthright and meticulous. I was really impressed with her computer skills among many other work-related attributes, and I told her so.

She replied, "I would be lost without you. Do you realize I come to your office and question you on so many applications and then, solely based on your knowledge, I simply get on the computer and just put it together? Once I have your input, the rest is easy for me."

"Really?"

"Yes, and furthermore, I sometimes follow you around the building watching and listening to how you interact with people. I'm trying to improve my personal relationships within the organization by emulating you. You're a master in public relations and a great role model for me to emulate."

"This may surprise you, but I actually like your many brat-like obstreperous mannerisms, so don't change too drastically, or you will lose your 'unusual charm.'"

"Gus, promise me that you'll never ever stop teasing me!"

"Amen!"

Actually, Charlotte's flattering comments were very moving. She was extremely bright and very proficient in discharging her duties. She knew how the pieces were to fit.

When I first arrived in Alaska, I worked very closely with our patient representative unit on a number of daily events. Financially speaking, this was a key area of concern for protecting the hospital against unnecessary loss of revenue due to laxity or imprudent management. Actually, it became very challenging to me to resolve certain incidents that arose relating to patient and financial situations.

I was asked to intercede on complicated issues, and also on many tenuous situations; for example, obtaining signatures on forms by reluctant spouses. Based on experience, these situations just need to be tactfully addressed.

To gain both recognition and their support, I willingly accepted every situation and was grateful that I was able to resolve them without difficulty. I asked their supervisor on several occasions if her staff was putting me on to see if I was adroit in solving their problems. Eventually, feeling the onus, they would say, "Don't ask him for his help—we will look like fools again."

They performed more independently at that point and considered me a good team player when appropriately needed. As time passed, their effectiveness was apparent to me and very reassuring, as this was a vital area of habitual challenge.

While I was working with this group, I was in my mid-fifties, while most of them were in their twenties and thirties—and they were all ladies. There were several nice places to go dancing in Anchorage, and, on a dare, they asked me to accompany them to one of them, which was featuring ballroom dancing. And they knew I could do the fast modern stuff, too. I went with them, and had a great time. Apparently, I made a hit on the dance floor with my ladies, and their guys also welcomed me to their group. They all wanted me to join them on a regular basis. My ladies said they would be on their best behavior and that they loved dancing with me. Actually, I mostly went alone, as I had so much fun with them—if I took a date of my own, the evening turned out more rigid and structured, and I felt less free to just get out there and go with the flow. (No offense to my regular date, however.)

The ladies separated work from fun and never ever took advantage of my after-hours friendship, as they were very respectful at all times. My relationship with this group of youngsters was a far cry from my relationship with my people during my regimented days at The Hospital of the Good Samaritan, where we had had to address a no-fraternization policy between management and staff. Richard somewhat impressively pointed out to me that I was on the "A list" in terms of being invited to all of the best parties in town. Lydia and I attended many parties in the very coldest weather—even in blizzards—but they were fun.

My colleagues at SJRMC continued to keep in touch with me. I would arrange to meet my inner circle for lunch when I returned to California each Christmas. One day, I received a fax from them pertaining to an open position at one of the specialty hospitals on the campus of the University of California at Los Angeles (UCLA). It was of interest to me, and I made arrangements to apply for the position. I informed the CFO at Providence Hospital of my interest when I asked for a few days off to travel to California. I spent about four hours meeting with the UCLA key personnel in the interview process. During this process, some of the people just came in and stayed long enough to cover their individual interests or areas of concerns.

After the meeting and spending some time alone with the human resources specialist, I asked, "What is your honest assessment of my performance?"

She said, "If you don't get this position, I'll be shocked. You answered all of their questions and presented yourself very capably."

I didn't know it at the time, but while I was returning to Alaska, a candidate with a solid background similar to that required by the open position was given the job. It wasn't until a few days after I'd returned to Alaska that I learned that I had come in second place because the chosen candidate had prior specific experience. I felt rather disappointed.

When I returned to Providence, and before I knew about the outcome at UCLA, I met the CFO and stated, "The position is still pending; I am awaiting UCLA's final decision."

He nonchalantly remarked, "I hope you decide to remain here and forget going south. However, as your plans are unsettled and, as I am working on our departmental budgets, I didn't put through an increase in your salary."

During the long winter months, I had worked at least ten hours each Saturday and Sunday, plus ten or more hours each weekday. I had been at my job for almost four years, and I believe I had worked, conservatively speaking, an additional eighteen months in just extra hours without remunerative consideration. I was management. I wanted to get my areas of responsibility first rate and just simply give of myself. It was just part of the job and part of fulfilling my responsibilities. To me, no conflict was involved. My priority was to successfully manage and maintain high standards within my departments. Making progress was my gratification—not remuneration.

After his comments he abruptly left my office. Regardless, of the outcome from the pending position at UCLA, I made a decision and said to myself (tunefully), "California here I come, right back where I started from!"

My near four years at Providence Hospital were definitely the most challenging years in healthcare for me personally. Had I not had a strong background based on my many years at The Hospital of the Good Samaritan and St. John's

Regional Medical Center, I would never have been able to cope with the ongoing challenges I faced at Providence. Virtually every basic procedure in my areas of responsibility had to be reexamined and reinforced. It took two years before I could take a deep breath knowing that constructive progress was being made and everyone was working in unison to achieve a common goal. When I had first arrived, I had had no idea what almost insurmountable opportunities were awaiting me.

Fortunately, being single and living great distances from family and friends, I was able to give the job everything I had to offer. My only family obligation was a promise to return home for the Christmas holidays. I fulfilled that obligation yearly.

Before I left Anchorage, Richard and his wife drove me all around that city pointing out the beautiful sights and telling me to stay. I made it a fun joy ride with them that day, but said that I must return to California. It was absolutely appropriate that I spend that time with them. Richard was pleased with my performance at Providence and he had been so encouraging to me during those difficult years. I made no mention to him of the CFO's comments about my salary.

While the challenges had been many, I had truly enjoyed my stay in Alaska and I have many fond memories, both personal and work-related to cherish. I met many wonderful and interesting people and had some great times being with them.

And, as a basically modest person, I am truly proud of my personal contribution to Providence Hospital. I implemented and achieved important procedures and provided great leadership and direction to my staff—all based on my bread-and-butter approach of working in the trenches with my co-workers. Teamwork!

I was very excited to reunite with my family, friends, and colleagues in Southern California. My journey and experiences in Alaska had, overall, been very challenging and fulfilling. So many wonderful people there opened their hearts and offered hospitality to me. I am so happy that I spent nearly four years in Alaska; they truly enriched my life. The wonderful people of Alaska, plus the beautiful state, greatly enhanced my journey from beginning to end. It was fabulous and, scenery-wise, a breathtaking experience. Back to the lower forty-eight!

21

After almost four years in Alaska, I returned to Los Angeles. I had a scheduled interview for a position at a large medical center in west Los Angeles the following day. While in Alaska, I had done some preliminary work toward obtaining this position, but, for some unknown reason, I had some dubious thoughts about applying. However, I tried to keep an open mind, even though I had that unexplainable gut feeling.

In meeting with the person that I would be reporting to, I experienced further scepticism about having a good working relationship. I had some other unfounded negative concerns and simply discarded any thought of working there. I did not reveal my thoughts, but I believe that, during our conversations, my interviewer detected my feelings of indifference. I plead guilty to transparency. I appeared noncommittal in pursuing the position. The end result was that they selected a candidate from within their facility. Paradoxically, the interviewer asked if he could submit my resume to their corporate office for other considerations. I declined his kind gesture. I really pondered over the thought that I may have inaccurately misjudged him. He had pessimistically discussed the woes confronting his hospital, showing me that he was incompatible with me and his nature was foreign to my very positive nature.

As I had just returned to California, I had mixed feelings, with a nonchalant temporary stage, about where to locate and what to do. My friend, the assistant CFO when I had been at SJRMC, had moved on from SJRMC, but we had stayed in touch. He advised me not to apply for a hospital position. He suggested that I become independent and work as a consultant. He and I had leadership associates in a prestigious consulting firm and I did seriously ponder over his valid suggestion to contact that organization for a consulting position.

One of our SJRMC sister hospitals had an open position and I knew the person leaving. Unaware of the prevalent issues, I felt somewhat awkward in applying for his position. Also, I was not too keen on some of the reporting issues. I met with their marketing folks who had a "front-burner" bone of contention with their information system regarding obtaining certain crucial information. I knew the key solution, but deferred from commenting. It simply applied to the use of a three-digit indicator. My reply/input may have had a negative implication on my counterpart. Dismissing further elaboration, I applied only to pacify the executive recruiter, who had worked with me originally on the UCLA position.

However, in addressing and contemplating resettlement considerations, I learned of an open position for a director of business services at the Delano Regional Medical Center in Delano, California. The hospital is located thirty miles north of Bakersfield, which would be acceptable to me. I also learned that their vice president of finance had just recently accepted her position at this hospital. She had previously been with Mercy Hospital in Bakersfield, which was a sister hospital to SJRMC. When I was at SJRMC, I had periodically visited Mercy Hospital.

I was staying with my sister in Woodland Hills on the outskirts of Los Angeles, and I drove to Delano and met with the VP. We instantly developed a good rapport, both having formerly worked with the Sisters of Mercy.

I believed that it would be challenging to work for a smaller hospital—and a great experience should I decide to become self-employed as a consultant. Also, the price of real estate was so moderate compared to the prices in the Los Angeles and Ventura areas that I decided to accept the position. So, the reasons were twofold.

The person at Mercy who had the same position that I had had at SJRMC, who had known me for years, passed on her kind thoughts to the VP. She was very happy to learn that I was contemplating moving to the Bakersfield area.

It seems that Murphy (and his law) had reappeared to greet me on the hospital steps. I was not surprised to learn that the hospital had recently gone through a computer conversion! The conversion had been done by an organization of which I knew nothing. Fortunately, a self-employed specialist, who represented the company, did the installation and remained as a consultant until all of the bugs were worked out. Literally and unbelievably, this never happens normally in the real business world. Through his guidance and applications, I quickly learned the new system. He was an incredible person to work with and we developed a good working and personal relationship. It was an anomaly to be afforded the ongoing assistance and the expertise of that specialist for an indefinite period of time. He had a wonderful wife who had sung on Broadway and who successfully underwent a liver transplant—a very exceptional and loving couple.

Due to the conversion and other departmental issues, patient accounts needed a lot of work. The hospital was privately owned by an individual who was personally interested in the day-to-day operation of the facility. There was a good administrator in place. Apart from patient accounts and related issues, the organization seemed to function well. Their accounts receivable had increased during the conversion and the emphasis was to reduce it to a satisfactory level. In terms of my responsibilities, the issues involved were mundane and solvable.

Shortly after I started working at the hospital, the owner and his entourage arrived for a meeting. The owner mentioned that he needed to understand why there were certain problems and what needed to be done. I frankly stated that I didn't have to ask anyone what needed to be done. I knew exactly what the problems were and the necessary steps to bring forth the solutions. I made these comments during the meeting and I assumed they were interpreted as efficacious and not as effrontery. The following day, the administrator informed me that the owner had requested a fax from me that day before 5 PM stating what steps were needed to solve our problems. In compliance, I prepared a comprehensive report on what steps needed to be taken and what enhancements were necessary for us to function proficiently.

Upon receipt of my request, the owner, without question, approved my complete report. Certain billing and other enhancements had to be initiated to fulfill our objectives. Also, I became more actively involved with certain other departments, such as medical records, to fulfill some of our billing needs to achieve our goals.

Fortunately, the computer specialist was still providing onsite services, and he helped me to fulfill the necessary computer applications. I was also involved in our utilization review department and worked with a wonderful licensed vocational nurse who was the supervisor. She also proficiently contributed to our efforts to expedite the completion of our billing trail to fulfill intermediary requirements. In conjunction with medical records and utilization review, I developed a close working relationship with our medical staff and their office employees, in the fulfillment of chart completion, attestations, and so forth. That was a challenging feat, as the medical staff vociferously informed me, upon my entry to the hospital, that they loathed the business office and spoke of it in disparaging terms.

Some physicians' offices were having reimbursement problems with their intermediaries. I volunteered my assistance and expertise and my involvement had a very positive impact. We were in a small community and my octopus-like behavior in assisting was appreciated and reciprocated by the medical staff and their employees. I stopped by their offices throughout the week to discuss mutual concerns. I was also involved in social services, risk management, and our patient representative unit, who were all tied into the same goals and objectives.

Those folks in these units reported to me. They worked independently and were knowledgeable and contributed to our overall team effort to reduce our accounts receivable to a satisfactory level.

As part of the program, the administrator asked that I be prepared to furnish a monthly report that specifically addressed revenues we could expect weekly. I had a slight trepidation in the preparation of that report; however, frankly to my surprise, I was totally on (or slightly over) target every single month.

I realized that any funding we required we had to initiate internally. We had neither endowments nor programs for additional sources of revenue. It was challenging and actually the reason I enjoyed being there. Needless to say, the VP and administrator were very pleased with our results. The assistant to the VP, who was managing the accounting department, was absolutely astonished that I continued to make my monthly target. He was about thirty-four years old and somewhat socially withdrawn until he started receiving my on-target monthly revenue reports—then he befriended me and shared my excitement. I was just damn lucky, as the only time I had walked on water was when I was in Alaska—and that was because it was frozen!

There is a large ventilation unit at Delano Regional Medical Center (DRMC), and several patients were referred to our hospital through a specialty company that contracted with our facility. The specialty organization searched for patients who required these services. In the process, they recruited many for our hospital, as we were so centrally located in our state.

For a small hospital, DRMC was very entrepreneurial and continued to seek other specialty and enhancement programs. This was very commendable for a small medical center in the heart of an agricultural community with a very limited commercial base.

While I was at DRMC, we went through a joint commission accreditation review. A team of physicians, nurses, and administrators came to review our standard practice manuals, patient and medical staff protocols, plus our plant and equipment to be certain that we were in compliance with licensing and other regulatory issues.

The licensed vocational nurse in utilization review and I worked together to write and revise our departmental procedure manuals for patient accounts, admitting and outpatient registration, along with utilization review, social services, risk management, and patient representatives. She purchased special binders and our reports looked absolutely, outstandingly professional. The incoming review team impressively gave us straight *A*'s for the finished product. Their recognition was gratifying, as they are not too keen in lavishing praise during the review process. They scrutinized key areas from top to bottom to be certain that the medical center was fulfilling the needs of the community and stood in compliance to their standards of excellence.

When we had similarly been reviewed at SJRMC, a member of the review team, while thumbing through our manual, asked if our patient representatives assisted persons with outpatient series concerns. I said, "Yes!" He asked if it was clearly stated in the procedural manual. Again, I responded, "Yes!" When he found the reference, his face lit up and, before leaving my office, said to the CFO, "I think he [pointing to me] is just about perfect." We both breathed a sigh of relief. That was my only personal involvement with a member of a review team.

When I started working at DRMC, I learned that many of my employees had family members who worked in agriculture and in the fields. During harvest time, they would bring me grapes and other fresh fruits. One lady asked, if she brought a crate of fruit for my family, could I arrange to take it to Woodland Hills on the weekend. Of course, I said I would. They were wonderful people, and it was such a treat after returning from Alaska to have so many fresh fruits and vegetables given to me. I, in turn, reciprocated by bringing unhealthy foods, such as sweet rolls, doughnuts, and tins of coffee, which they all devoured.

When I worked on the weekends, after work I would walk through the vineyards and look at the grapes growing, as well as the grapes stretched out on long rolls of paper basking in the sun turning into raisins. I love farming and agriculture. One of my supervisors mentioned that I had told her how I had loved picking cherries off of the trees when I was a youngster. She was wonderful. One day, with a deadpan expression on her face, she told me I was going to return to my youth on the following Saturday. I said, "What are you talking about?"

Said she, "You are going cherry picking with me." I picked forty or fifty pounds for her that Saturday—mostly from the upper branches as I stood on a ladder. It was fun, and certainly reminded me of my youth when I had climbed those trees—usually after a rainstorm—and eaten mostly Bing cherries.

I believe the owner of DRMC both liked and respected me. I surmised that he thought I was somewhat arrogant or opinionated or both, but he truly recognized my performance. I stayed at the hospital only for twenty months, and, just before I left, he stopped for an informal chat and included a little controversy. He said,

"You compute your days outstanding in gross days, whereas the trend is now in net days." I said, "I could agree with that formula. However, in computing in gross days and knowing by that method I had reduced the accounts receivable by fifty percent, the end result works for me."

"Touché!"

Some time after I left, the owner sold his interest in the hospital. Frankly, I gave high marks to the owner and the administrator as they really had set expectations for their management staff. In the process, they were innovative in bringing new programs and concepts onboard.

Before leaving, I put a comprehensive plan in place to retain the accounts receivable at an acceptable level. I was delighted to learn that they continued to maintain those good standards after my departure. I enjoyed my stay there; it was a great opportunity to work in a smaller hospital and in a less-populated community.

Shortly before my departure from DRMC, I planned a visit to see my Munro relatives in Ontario. I asked Michele to join me once more, with the proviso that she refrain from accepting any of our cousin's wonderful fruitcake. It was a difficult decision giving up another opportunity to do one of my imitations of her. She reluctantly agreed.

Cecil Inglehart was living in Toronto, and had been for many years. We had lost touch with each other after he left Vancouver. I located his telephone number and called him. "Hello, is this the Inglehart residence?"

A lady responded, "Yes."

"Am I speaking with Mrs. Cecil Inglehart?"

"Yes."

"I am an old family friend, originally from Vancouver, calling Cecil."

"He's home. I'll call him to the telephone. May I have your name, please?"

"Tell him it is Gus Munro."

"WHAT! You are THE Gus Munro?"

"I am he."

"Oh my goodness, he's going to be shocked and pleasantly surprised. I can't believe this is happening. We've never met, but I know all about you and your family. This is unbelievable! I'll call him to the telephone."

"Gus Munro, where the hell have you been all of these years? I am so happy to hear your voice. Where are you?"

"I am in California. My niece and I will be coming to Toronto to visit relatives—hopefully including you and your family."

"Gus, I keep telling my family there is one person in this world I want to see before I die, and that person is Gus Munro. Gus, my sister Rita lives within driving distance from us and she will be able to come to our reunion. She'll be so excited to know that you're coming. I'll get in touch with her right away." We continued our conversation about our reunion. It was an exciting experience for both of us, and it seemed the same for his wife, too.

Unfortunately, a difficult situation arose at the hospital regarding an intermediary issue that was so important I had to cancel our trip. The flight tickets and other arrangements had been made. I called my sister Marjorie to see if she would be interested in taking my place. She had never met our relatives and she agreed to the trip. Michele and Marjorie had a great visit, with Marjorie meeting our Munro family and Michele reacquainting with them. The Munro family was delighted to meet my sister and to see Michele once more and they had planned events to cover their brief stay in Ontario.

My sister spoke with Cecil and explained the situation. Unfortunately, due to time restraints they were unable to arrange a visit to see Cecil and his family.

This, unfortunately, is a good example of my dedication to my work and responsibilities, as I declined to go solely based on that important work issue. To me, it was critical that I remain at work—one of those unfortunate situations. When Cecil left for Toronto, those many years ago, I had no idea that, sadly, I would never ever see him again!

22

After twenty months at DRMC, I accepted a position at Orthopaedic Hospital in Los Angeles. I started working there in early June 1992. Years earlier, I had attended a meeting at that hospital. It had a good reputation and it had been primarily dedicated to serving the orthopaedic needs of children. They also provided adult services; however, the primary focus remained on their children's programs. The hospital also has a large hemophilia center, which had been initiated by fruition, as so many hemophiliacs required orthopaedic services. The hospital combined their treatment services in addressing both conditions simultaneously.

We had close family friends who had a son who was a haemophiliac. He received excellent treatment at this hospital for several years. The family was also treated admirably, and I was impressed with their favorable comments regarding the hospital. I always remembered the kind gestures afforded our family friends and viewed the hospital as commendable in pursuing their mission for both children and adults.

I accepted the position of director of business services and the admitting office, emergency room registration unit, and an extremely large outpatient admitting center primarily for children's services. I quickly learned that I would also to be deeply involved in the complexities of the financial affairs of our hemophilia patients. As this was a specialty hospital, our inpatient admissions were much lower than those of a full-service hospital. This was in part due to Managed Care that had to address the reductions in both the Medicare and Medicaid (Medi-Cal in California) programs. The private sector did not want the shifting of costs to them; thus, major insurance companies and intermediaries were negotiating preferentially with full-service hospitals. Additionally, many Medicare recipients were being encouraged to join plans offered by major insurance companies and medical groups, thus eliminating their co-payments and offering other considerations. However, under this arrangement, all services provided had to be within the membership network. Thus, Medicare patients had to waive their right to receive services at non-contracting medical facilities. Apart from other considerations, the advance of medical treatment reduced the orthopaedic inpatient hospital length of stay dramatically. The average length of stay was reduced to a range of from three to five days total hospital confinement.

When I started at the hospital I had a frank discussion with the CFO, who was both an attorney and CPA. It was imperative that we establish a comprehensive work plan. I came with excellent references, but I was sixty-one, and we were going under the assumption that I would probably retire at the customary age of sixty-five. Upon my retirement, the CFO was hopeful that we could elevate the current billing supervisor to assume my role. The billing supervisor had been with the hospital for many years and was actively involved in all phases of business and admitting services. These were preliminary discussions and, as a hands-on person, I would need to work with the people and the workflow and volumes before making any future plans or draw any conclusions. I needed to see and personally evaluate each employee.

I clearly detected that the CFO would put me through the test and make his own judgment as to my proficiency. He spoke with me very frankly, but he seemed to be heedful as he selected his words. I later learned that my assessment was correct. He had experienced some disagreements with others who had reported to him and, as a result, he put himself in a cautionary mode.

The CFO stated straightforwardly that the medical staff was not too enchanted with the business office and there was an immediate priority to improve that situation. As I mentioned previously, comments relating to the disgruntlement of the medical staff seemed to be ongoing and posed no threat to me. However, I learned that most of the physicians' offices were on campus, which I considered a windfall, and I told him so. Being in close proximity to the physician offices made it easy for me to stop by and introduce myself and get the wheels in motion.

The CFO was surprised when I informed him that I could establish a more favorable image with the medical staff offices within six weeks—unequivocally. He looked at me somewhat skeptically at my off-the-cuff remark, but made no challenging response to refute my assessment. I perceived that he was impressed by my assertiveness and probably thought the proof would be in the pudding. In assessing new persons, words and performance of "bosses" often differ.

I immediately ingratiated myself by popping into the various physicians' offices, introducing myself to staff members, and apologizing for barging in unannounced. I was graciously received, and I frankly asked that they share their concerns regarding the business office. I informed them that my goal was to immediately change the relationship between their offices and the business office. I also sent follow-up letters to them regarding their needs and expectations in the form of a questionnaire and freestyle request for input. This was intended to stimulate participation and open new avenues of communication. I also informed them that I was an active participant in resolving patient issues and was ready to personally serve their needs. This dialogue immediately became the beginning of a good rapport with both physicians and their staff. My style was to hit the basic bread-and-butter list.

We started addressing individual patient's specific needs. The physicians and their staff members soon realized that I was a positive member of the team—being both assertive and compromising in resolving issues. The CFO ebulliently informed me that the physicians and their staff were almost tripping him in the halls. They were telling him that they were making good progress with Gus Munro. There is nothing more reassuring than to receive direct feedback that positive results are manifesting and changing a bad situation.

My perception was that the CFO was quite brilliant, and he cogently expressed his thoughts and expectations. When I first arrived, he gave me some correspondence from three or four disgruntled patients and/or their representatives concerning the business office. I quickly responded to each person and resolved his or her situation and sent copies of my confirming correspondence to the CFO as a routine gesture. A quick response and follow-through are key elements in developing your presence within an organization to affirm participation and favorable team membership.

I was in the CFO's office one day, and he pulled from his desk drawer the copies of the letters I had sent. He informed me that he found my correspondence extremely well written. He thought my letters were written courteously, professionally, and appropriately, addressing the needs and concerns of our patients. He further stated that the way I had conducted myself in working with other departments had not gone unnoticed. He stated that he had received excellent feedback from my peers—which pleased me. He also reiterated his gratitude and admiration in my resolution of the ongoing problems relating to the negative relationship between the medical offices and the business office. He asserted that I had fulfilled my pledged assurance to him that it would be done expediently. He hinted gratefully that I had removed a troublesome burden from his shoulders.

I had been taken by his candor and astuteness, but thought he was somewhat shrewdly trying to measure my overall effectiveness. I could tell that he was tremendously impressed that I had effortlessly solved the physician office problem. However, I assumed I somehow came across as being somewhat self-effacing. I perceived he was sort of testing the water to see if I was plagued with any superficial tendencies, or if I could execute effectively anything assigned to me. Being in this position is not one of the joys of being the new kid on the block, so to speak!

I also surmised, and it was later confirmed, that, as assertive and as efficacious as he was in identifying the future needs of the hospital, there was a definite divisiveness among his group of directors and managers. He had been both challenging and critical in evaluating their performance, in terms of fulfilling both the hospital and the individual departmental objectives. That measurement was clearly included in each individual director or manager's annual evaluation. A few members of the management team were very disgruntled having received unsatisfactory performance evaluations. During the monthly management meetings, they took the opportunity to fire innuendoes in his direction when discussing expectations. Those of us on the sidelines quickly discerned when the game was in action—CFO verses disgruntled manager or director. The CFO was a fair and levelheaded person and no intellectual slouch. Regardless of the controversy and shaded ill will, he tenaciously stayed exactly on course, which I most admired. He was tough.

He requested that I consider making a concerted effort in downsizing to reduce my staffing complement both by eliminating certain positions and by obtaining no replacements when attrition occurred. My background had been in running a tight ship regarding staffing complements, and his thoughts were akin to mine. As part of our encompassing discussion, I informed him that my areas of responsibility were far less than anticipated. With a low inpatient census, I needed additional duties to increase my workload to a much higher level. I offered my services to pick-up the slack in some other areas within the hospital.

I was used to working in much larger hospitals than both Orthopaedic Hospital and DRMC, with very heavy inpatient volumes. I had been involved in public relations activities, marketing, and other promotional services, and special assignments.

Around that time, a female patient was admitted with an acute acquired condition normally exhibited by males only. The constant care and supplies for this patient were horrendous and our costs were astronomical. Our anticipated reimbursement under this patient's insurance plan was less than paltry.

I immediately challenged the insurance carrier through both their internal legal representatives and their medical review department, with complete medical documentation and supporting charges and costs involved for special products and supplies, requesting commensurate reimbursement. This was a difficult case, and I spent a great deal of time and effort pursuing this claim. Because of the extreme illness and circumstances, we were equitably reimbursed.

The CFO was astonished that I had been able to resolve the claim so equitably and amicably myself with the insurance carrier without some legal assistance.

During that period, I worked on a couple of similar difficult cases involving other insurance carriers that I addressed in the same manner. It was almost bewildering to the CFO that I had been so successful. While the reimbursements were appropriately justifiable, I was extremely pleased with the outcome as those three cases more than covered my salary for the next six or seven years. Modestly I can say that, over the years, I had resolved many such cases.

A young man named Robert was in charge of occupational therapy. He stopped by my office with a proposal. He asked if I could assist him and his department to relocate to an identified vacant space in the hospital. His current department was located in one of our satellite buildings. His request to relocate was predicated on being in closer proximity to serve those patients who were hospitalized. I was convinced that it could be a positive move, and I discussed it with the CFO, who gave me the green light.

To fulfill this plan, we needed to raise funds through our Women's Guild. The therapist and I met with the guild director and she approved the funds. In a short period of time, the unit was ready for occupancy and all of our goals had been achieved. The therapist and I met to discuss our closing issues. I said, "Before the open house, I want you to write a nice thank you letter to the guild director for approving the allocation of funds to cover this project."

"Gus, how do I write a thank you letter?"

"Good night, do I have to do everything?"

"I am a 'hands-on' therapist, with no experience in writing thank you letters. Help!"

"Okay, I'll write the letter for your signature. This is very important, not only for etiquette, but we may need some more help down the road."

During open house, the guild director (a good colleague, by the way) pulled me aside for conversation. "Gus, Robert sent me one of the nicest thank you letters I ever received. I was so pleased with his comments, so beautifully written. It was a wonderful letter."

"I am pleased that he sent you a nice letter," said I, with crossed fingers. Then I went to find Robert. "Robert, the guild director said that your thank you letter to her was wonderful."

Laughingly, he said, "Gus, did you tell her that I have an excellent secretary?"

"Yeah, sure. I did the work and you got the glory."

Shortly thereafter, the director of medical records took ill and required major surgery and an extended period for her recuperation. She and I had become fast friends when I joined the hospital. Together we had promoted and conducted some luncheons for our hospital staff and the medical staff offices located on campus. They were procedural and educational programs, informally conducted, and they further enhanced internal relationships. We also had worked together on some other promotional projects for third-party payers and others regarding our services as well.

Unfortunately, her surgery revealed that she was seriously ill and required ongoing medical care and treatment. Sadly, her prognosis was not encouraging. In making arrangements for an extended leave of absence she requested that the CFO assign her duties to me as an interim solution. She knew elsewhere, I had worked closely with medical records on special projects. The additional responsibilities eliminated the work vacuum that I had been experiencing. I was happy to assist and support my colleague during this period of need.

Sadly, the director of medical records passed away after a short few months of convalescent care. She was a wonderful lady and, tragically, still very young. It was so sad for her husband and family and the rest of us, too. In reorganizing the department, I recommended that the manager of utilization review, who was a registered nurse and long-term care manager, be promoted as director of both departments. My suggestion was approved, and the new director hired an excellent medical records specialist to manage the medical records department under her direction.

Thereafter, I was assigned to and accepted some of the duties that had been fulfilled by a vice president who was leaving the hospital. Those duties included marketing and contracting issues—for the hospital and also for some of our medical staff. In accepting the additional responsibilities, I became directly involved in working with our physicians and in trying to promote more patient referrals for them as a group. I had to restructure my duties in the business office to accommodate the marketing and contracting responsibilities. And further, I had to allow for cold calling "introductory solicitation" telephone time during the day in my efforts to attempt to generate more business.

I met with the CFO and informed him that I would assume all of the preparatory contracting work with the proviso that he approve and endorse all contracts. He heartily agreed for the hospital, and allowed me to work with the physicians on their contracts as well. I was to attend my first meeting after being assigned to participate in marketing/contracting with the medical group. I had completed a twelve-page report on my activities for the month. I listed all of my cold calling to attract new business, insurance companies for new contracts, and, through researching our Workers' Compensation financial class, identified the individuals who had sent patients to us through our medical staff.

In preparing the listing and summary, I indicated key persons and their telephone numbers. At this point, I had very limited experience with our medical staff on marketing issues per se. I asked the CFO to review my report to be certain it was meaningful and hopefully to demonstrate that I had been actively engaging sufficient time to this new project. He thought the report was comprehensive and demonstrated that I was cognizant of what needed to be achieved. The meeting went well and the physicians reviewed my report in a nonjudgmental manner. One physician kept encircling certain data in red and I couldn't discern whether that was a negative or positive exercise. His office assistant said later that it was positive.

During the meeting I informed the medical staff that I needed suitable brochures and other documentation to distribute to my contacts. Without adequate material, my hands were semi-tied in trying to promote our services. The physician who had been drawing the red ink circles quickly injected that I was absolutely right. He further stated that I needed to be furnished with effective promotional material for both physician and hospital services to expand our patient referral base.

After that meeting, I immediately befriended Dr. Gordon, an anesthesiologist who represented our anesthesia group practice and who was also president of our medical group. In working with various medical groups and other third-party payers, he actively assisted me in addressing physician-related issues. He helped me enormously in trying to generate new business. After my initial marketing contacts, he stopped by my office on a daily basis offering assistance and providing encouragement. He was vehemently interested in forging ahead.

Shortly thereafter, the CFO left the hospital to relocate in the Midwest. I must confess that I was saddened by his departure. He quintessentially epitomized my image of an outstanding CFO. We had developed a great rapport and he was challenging to report to. We shared concurrent ongoing objectives for my departments and the medical center.

Judging from my final yearly evaluation, the feeling was mutual. I apparently received the highest evaluation among those reporting to him. My report card, which he prepared close to his departure, was somewhat surprising, but appreciated.

His adroitness and moral standards were equally distributed. He was a great family man and professionally received many accolades, both within the hospital and from the outside. He was highly regarded by peers in other medical centers, who periodically attended special association meetings in our hospital.

On an interim basis, the hospital president, Dr. Luck, assumed many of the responsibilities for that position until it was filled. To further assist me, Dr. Luck hired a consultant to manage our contracting for both hospital-and physician-related business. Her name was Sue, and she was a treasure to the hospital and to me. She and our organization instantaneously fit like a glove.

Sue was extremely forthright in conducting and discharging her affairs, both internally and externally, on all management levels. Unbeknownst to her, that was part of her charm. We became a great team in addressing hospital and physician issues—or else we were damn lucky, as on any given situation our separate or combined knowledge or experience were our steadfast tools of resolution. Perhaps it was a little of both, as we always seemed to pull a good result out of the hat, so to speak. We were able to generate many new contracts and increase volumes from those in place covering both physician and hospital services.

In the business office, my wonderful assistant, Mattie, was extremely knowledgeable—a very hardworking lady who was blessed with a good sense of humor. She was a delightful partner. I truly admired her work ethic and she represented a perfect standard in the management and utilization of her time.

I loved teasing her. As I assessed her thoughts on people and other issues, including work gossip, I realized she was somewhat wholesomely and refreshingly naive and strongly identified with and was devoted to the goodness of her church and congregation. On one occasion, during a teasing episode, her retort to my comment was, "Do you think I fell off of a turnip truck yesterday?"

I replied, "No, probably the day before!"

She told her two adult children those comments—and I think they laughingly agreed with me. She said they teased her all weekend, "Probably the day before, Mother!"

Before the CFO left the hospital, he executed the return of our physician billing services from a private organization. Both Mattie and I worked with him, and, through her recommendation, acquired the services of a physician billing computer organization to reestablish our in-house services. She assumed full responsibility in reestablishing the physician billing services as a unit within the business office. She and I worked together in designating our individual responsibilities within our departments and it worked out well.

Aside from my departmental activities, I assumed other administrative duties during an interim period when there were two open positions for both a chief operating officer and a chief financial officer. Our board of directors was also developing and negotiating the feasibility of an alignment with another medical facility to eventually discontinue our inpatient services on site, because of our diminishing inpatient volumes. This would be a gigantic undertaking, with many ramifications to consider. Thus, the idea needed to be sagaciously explored and discreetly planned in stages.

The hospital was blessed with a solid foundation that enabled the fulfillment of our mission to the care and treatment of children. During this transitional period, the foundation received, unexpectedly, a wonderful gift of about $25,000,000. A lady who had lived in the San Fernando Valley expired and left this generous legacy to Orthopaedic Hospital and similar and/or varied amounts to other medical centers. This benefactor had owned a very modest tract home in North Hollywood and lived unpretentiously, socializing with her neighbors by having dinner with them at their local Denny's coffee shop on Saturday night. Her grandfather had acquired Kellogg's Corn Flakes stock, which had been passed down to her and which increased over the years, making her a wealthy lady. Her net worth was in the millions. Apparently she had a doll collection, but, other than that, lived a very unaffected lifestyle. This generous donation greatly enhanced our foundation and somewhat deferred the immediacy of having to swiftly negotiate to fulfill our inpatient services at another medical center. However, unions with other medical centers still sat on the back burner for consideration.

The hospital acquired a new but seasoned chief operations officer, Anora, who was great and eventually eliminated the necessity of my part-time involvement in working on special administrative projects. Later, the hospital hired a new CFO, Jeffrey, a young man who was a Harvard graduate and also had a law degree from UCLA.

I was elated to learn that, in the sunset of my healthcare career, I would be finally working with a Harvard man, which had been one of my long-term desires. I must preface the exclusion of members of the medical staff whom I worked with over the years who may have attended Harvard. Strangely, as a grade-school dropout, I believed a most fulfilling and epitomizing experience would be to work in tandem with a Harvard graduate—both ends of the spectrum working together. That would be the icing on the cake, so to speak, to my career. Before meeting with him, I learned that he would be wearing two hats: CFO and legal counsel in negotiating our transitional activities for the provision of inpatient services and other alliances elsewhere. These were very challenging responsibilities for this new hire to fulfill.

Jeffrey was twenty-eight years old, above average height, slim, dark haired, very good looking, and impeccably dressed. He looked like a Mr. GQ and could easily have graced that magazine or *Esquire*. He spoke both articulately and commandingly, and he was extremely gracious and cordial to me. I perceived he was cautiously attempting to measure both my proclivities and abilities simultaneously. Aside from my impression, with all of those overwhelming attributes, there was only one problem—he and I just didn't seem to "jell."

In meeting with Jeff, for some reason I developed a somewhat confrontational attitude toward him. I dismissed any thoughts of attempting to develop a rapport with him. In retrospect, I can blame myself, as I seemed to have had an inexplicable and unrealistic personal expectation of working with this young Harvard man who came long overdue into my life—but quite unexpectedly. He was subjected to my close scrutiny. Aside from the BS, I unconsciously recognized his good qualities.

To complete the picture, like me, he was blessed with boundless energy and he would stop by the local gym at the crack of dawn most mornings for a routine workout. He would arrive to work laden down with all of his gym paraphernalia or arrive earlier in gym clothing to work before heading for the gym. He was extremely motivated, compulsive, and unstinting in fulfilling his daily workout regiment. I was to learn much later that, aside from his position and background, he was, in his own perception, just a plain, regular guy, totally unpretentious and very comfortable in his surroundings. He leaped at fulfilling prescribed expectations.

After meeting with Jeff, I went back to Anora and said, "I cannot nickname him 'Super Brat,' as John McEnroe has that title. I shall have to settle mundanely for 'Boy Wonder.'" Needless to say, this was total idiocy and immaturity on my part. Anora tried to pacify me by saying that I was jumping the gun in assessing him and that I needed to work with him and to try and develop a better rapport.

She further stated that Jeff had a lot to offer our hospital. She found him very bright and affable, and she felt he would bring forth positive results in executing his responsibilities at our hospital. She also emphasized the critical need for his legal expertise in the necessary transitional changes both internally and externally. Additionally, he had come highly recommended, and Dr. Luck was extremely impressed with this very well-educated young man.

After my third meeting with him, I thought, *"This isn't going to work for us."* By that time, I had reached sixty-five years old, and I decided to leave the following spring. Meanwhile, Jeff started discreetly working with Mattie on our physician billing unit and other related issues. I reported to him on the business office, and we met each week. There seemed to be a semi-postponement in negotiating inpatient services elsewhere, thus affording Jeff the opportunity to become very heavily involved and well informed in all departments under his directorship—such as information systems and others to improve the workflow.

When spring arrived and I contemplated retirement, I was asked to remain with the hospital and, by choice, I transferred to the marketing department to continue my work there. Meanwhile, Anora asked if I wanted to become the director of marketing. I declined and she hired a young woman named Chris for that position. To best fit my needs to continue, I joined Sue as a consultant working in the marketing department and reporting directly to Dr. Luck.

Before leaving the business office, I had met with Anora and Chris on Chris's second interview, at which time Anora informed Chris that I had been offered the marketing position but declined it. When Chris came onboard, I worked closely and supportively with her. At the end of her first week, she pointing to me and said, "My possible enemy has turned out to be my best friend." When I joined Chris, Mattie assumed my role in patient accounts as we had originally planned.

In the process, Jeff and I developed a cordial relationship. He was very supportive and instrumental in seeing that I was favorably resituated in marketing as a consultant. That seemed to be of paramount importance to him. What I did not see immediately was the fact that Jeff and I were very much alike. I was astonished at the similarities in the way we both addressed and discharged our duties. I found it to be somewhat of a strange correlation and comparison between a dropout and Harvard graduate. We both started our week on Sunday and both worked long hours.

By my observation, Jeff was an octopus—involved in everything and leaving no stone untouched. Had I been in his position in coming to Orthopaedic Hospital, I would have developed the same work structure that he established.

In essence, what I didn't realize at the time was that he had given me a confirmation of what I had been doing singly myself over the years. While we functioned differently in our respective positions, after my departure from the business office, he assumed some of the exact audit trails that I had used, purely on his own volition. Again, the similarity to our method of operation and basic functions seemed uncanny. We both just quietly did what it took to get the job done.

Quite truthfully, Jeff is the person I have worked with who is closest to myself in terms of style and executing the work. I have marveled at his subdued tenacity as he pursued and fulfilled his duties and responsibilities within the organization so effortlessly. On the day of the monthly meeting of the board of directors, he was always in at the crack of dawn, around 5 AM, to perform a diligent last-minute review. The same standard applied in meeting with the business office for a review of accounts receivable. He had the same meticulous criteria because everything counted equally with him. He worked methodically but unpretentiously, laboring in the corporate trenches and getting good results.

Jeff's established work performance criteria were exactly the same as mine by example. Unbeknownst to him, he gave this grade-school dropout both vindication and validation for my performance over the years.

Before I run ahead of myself, here is some catch-up on the Jeff story. I was staying in west Los Angeles during the week and he asked for a ride home one afternoon. He was to meet his fiancée at his apartment and he asked me to stop by a corner florist shop before we reached his apartment.

While I waited for him in the car, I recalled having stopped by the same floral company years before, to buy flowers for my wife. When we met Jeff's fiancée Marissa, an extremely attractive and gracious young lady, in front of the apartment building, he presented her with a rose and introduced me as his good friend, Gus. I thought at the time, *I bet she has heard some horrible tales about me.* Jeff's performance and introduction was touching.

As I drove away, I thought that I needed to revisit my feelings about Jeff. I may have misjudged him—either that or he had just given me the Academy Award performance of his life. I decided I had misjudged him. It also occurred to me that, on a regular working relationship basis, I could have simply been wrong. He was a good guy and I should have left it at that.

One day, I casually mentioned to his secretary, "Where is Jeff?" She said that he and Marissa were vacationing in Paris. I suddenly thought, *Suppose he moves on somewhere else?* I suddenly became very emotional and realized I had to reassess my thoughts about him. I realized that I had misjudged him. He was a very capable and innovative person and he had done an outstanding job for the hospital—in all of his departments. Also, I had to consider all of the legal issues relating to the transition. I sagaciously admitted to myself that I was not only appreciative of his work performance, but I admired him very much. And I had personally become very fond of him through quiet observation.

When he returned from Paris I set up a personal meeting with him. Needless to say, after dealing with this bombastic Scorpio, he was surprised and delighted in conversing with the real me. He temporarily may have questioned my sincerity, but we soon became very close and we remained that way for several years. After performing brilliantly at the hospital, he decided to concentrate on his law career and went with a major national organization. I was extremely upset about his leaving, and Anora prudently put me in charge of his farewell party so that I could concentrate on the more positive aspects. After he had settled into his new position, he and I had dinner one night and he informed me that he and Marissa were going to wed.

We had a father-and-son type of evening. I showered him with heartfelt complimentary statements on what a wonderful person he truly was and he, when leaving, asked that I convey those nice thoughts to Marissa. I did, but it wasn't necessary. She already knew all of his wonderful attributes.

They are very happily married and reside in a beautiful home in the Pasadena hills with their little daughter and Marissa's son from a prior marriage. Jeff is a wonderful husband and father and so devoted to them and to his mother and other members of his family. To me, that Harvard guy was worth waiting for, as he turned out to be so very special. My feelings for him are inexplicable. Apart from his wonderful qualities he is, conversely, also a "handful"—constantly challenging me and simultaneously taking great pleasure in doing so.

For a brilliant young man, he has been blessed abundantly with brat-like qualities toward me. I assume that it is sort of like payback time from his prospective, regarding our earlier confrontational "frontier days." When he finally sorted this situation out in his methodical way, it seemed he decided what he had to do to accept me into his inner circle.

He let bygones be bygones. He came up with the most reprehensible, heinous, and unconscionable solution that has placed me in an untenable position. So what horrendous act has befallen on me? *Jeffrey has become my father!* Due to my now somewhat precarious and subservient status, I have thus been phasing into a mellowing process. I just simply agree with what he says and wink at Marissa if I have a divergent opinion. However, on a brighter note, one evening, outside a restaurant where we had all shared a delicious meal, I embraced both Marissa and Jeffrey and we spoke some parting words. After they left, the parking attendant said to me, "I can tell that young man is your son."

I said, "He is the son I never had!"

Said he, "Same thing!"

Not really, but I loved his observation and comments!

23

On the marketing front, I still needed to have more brochures and material available for distribution. Fortunately, when Chris came aboard, she immediately focused on our need for printed material and did an encompassing job in sufficiently fulfilling our needs. In preparing our print material, Chris worked closely with Dr. Luck, Dr. Gordon, and others in bringing the material together. Due to Chris's good work, our marketing packages, complete with brochures, were outstandingly prepared. We received many favorable comments from the recipients.

She and I worked together and strengthened our referral system internally and externally. It was a great benefit to our medical staff and the providers and the patients involved. Chris also provided ongoing workshops internally and externally for case managers—addressing the needs of Workers' Compensation category patients.

My final years in marketing were a great joy. I was able to work very closely with all hospital departments, medical offices, third-party payers, and, most importantly, many individual patients as I addressed their special needs.

I spent a total of eleven years almost to the day at Orthopaedic Hospital. It was a great experience and I still remain very close to the organization. They recently have constructed a new building to further accommodate their children's programs. They also recently constructed a new school. It is now open on their campus to accommodate students majoring in science. They are very excited about the establishment of this facility, along with their science programs.

Currently, in conjunction with their affiliation with UCLA, the hospital is erecting a new building at the Santa Monica location to accommodate the move of inpatient services to that facility. Exciting things are happening for this medical center in the next few years that will be a great benefit to the community.

At the time I started working at Orthopaedic Hospital, my niece Robin was pregnant for the first time. One weekend, upon returning from Bakersfield to start the working week, I stopped by to see Robin and her husband Paul. Paul asked me to join them on a stroll along the beach at Santa Monica. The subject of our beach conversation was the selection of a name for the soon-to-be-born son. I wanted a Scottish name, free from nicknames, such as Ian or Ross. However, as merely the great uncle I was soon to be voted out. Paul emphatically requested the name Kyle—also not prone to nicknaming. Robin and I relented to the wish of a forthcoming father expecting his first son. During our stroll, I also committed myself to being an active babysitter—pointing out that this would be our first new family member to be born in about twenty-five years.

Along with members of both families, we happily greeted Kyle by gazing at him in the observation-type medical unit. He had just received an injection in his foot and he had a tear running down his face. I commiserated with all of the pain involved in being a newborn, but also immediately loved this beautiful little baby. Before assuming my role as part-time babysitter so that Robin could return to work, I initially joined Paul and baby to begin with to learn the basic steps of infant care. Thankfully, Paul had already taken a quick course in infant care.

Paul's mother had a large deluxe apartment in Brentwood. I gave up my small rental apartment in Brentwood to resettle in her home during the working week. Paul worked days and Robin worked the afternoon shift. As I worked days during the week, I had the flexibility of working out my schedule to include Kyle. It was fun for Paul's mother and me to share Kyle. He had an excellent babysitter and I arranged to pick him up at her home a couple of late afternoons during the week. We must have done a good job, as three years later our workload was doubled with the birth of Grant, their second son. I have a very close relationship with my great nephews as we bonded very early.

During my years staying with Paul's mother Lucy in Brentwood, the murder of Nicole Brown Simpson took place, followed by the O.J. Simpson trial. The murder scene was two blocks from our apartment. My routine evening walk took me by the victim's condominium. It was constantly plagued with crowds of sightseers for months and months. One evening I met a neighbor who had been a friend to both Simpsons, and she informed me that they had had what she called a love-hate relationship.

On a curious note, the father and stepmother of President Clinton's love interest, Monica Lewinsky, resided in Brentwood three or four blocks from our apartment. We had more than our share of sightseers canvassing the neighborhood covering these places of media interest that only added to our already congested traffic.

Here is a very brief update on my young friend Robert from Alaska whom I had identified as having great potentialities: Robert worked at a large New Jersey hospital for several years as a director and he became president of an eastern chapter of admitting directors. He later became a vice president of a healthcare-related computer company and he has done extremely well. In my experience, he is the standard bearer for people who work their way through the ranks. I am so proud of him and what he has achieved. He has also been an exemplary husband and father, and, to me, a great friend. He has great writing skills and he needs to put his work experience on paper. He tells everyone that I was his mentor—and to refute his remarks is like turning down my favorite dessert (crème brûlée)!

I had the pleasure of reporting to Dr. Luck, who is president of Orthopaedic Hospital and their foundation and medical staff. He also maintains his own private practice on campus. His father, also an orthopaedic physician had retired from active practice before I started working at our hospital. The father had devoted his lifetime career to the hospital. He was instrumental in initially developing and expanding adult programs to complement those already in place. Their key focus was providing full orthopaedic services through the children's programs. However, the adult programs enhanced the overall mission of the hospital. Dr. Luck, as heir apparent, was destined to assume the leadership of the hospital, along with the other entities and affiliations that are based on the downtown campus or elsewhere.

Aside from full orthopaedic services, Dr. Luck also specializes in the treatment and care of hemophilia patients. The hospital is an established hemophilia center and Dr. Luck is totally responsible for orthopaedic care for both inpatient and outpatient services. These patients are commonly prone to suffering with severe knee problems. He performs a special outpatient knee procedure for those patients that qualify, in lieu of a total knee replacement surgery. Patients come from all parts of this country for the procedure—which he has been doing successfully for so many years.

Needless to say, among his many responsibilities involving the hospital, medical staff, foundation, and his private practice, he is extremely busy and must manage his time sagaciously to coincide with a very busy schedule. Apart from being an excellent physician and surgeon, he is a great humanitarian and extremely meticulous in fulfilling patient needs. He quickly identified my interest and compassion concerning the needs of our patients. He and I soon initiated an informal and very active special working relationship.

I worked closely with his private and administrative office. In any patient situations requiring my intervention relating to insurance, financial issues, or logistics, he simply would say, "Call Gus and get him involved." When needing his assistance, I would look for him in the parking lot (as I knew when he arrived), in the hemophilia unit on his assigned days, in the hallways, or in his office. When I caught him on the run, he knew that I would not keep him long from his activities, or confront him with any time-consuming extemporaneous topics.

Dr. Luck was the only person with whom I had such a unique working relationship. Our ongoing discussions on the run became perfectly normal to both of us. We both seemed to share the same values, loyalties, and confidentialities, and felt very comfortable in working together. Although he did think I was opinionated! Three out of four isn't bad! Occasionally, I would find it necessary to catch up with him in his busy clinic in the hemophilia unit. If I found him surrounded by medical professionals, along with patients and their family members, I would leave. I soon learned, however, if I needed him urgently, that I should just remain semi-conspicuously on the edge of activity. He would spot me between patients and firing off dictation or instructions, and he would say, "What do you need?" I have always marveled at his meticulous inherent protocol.

In working in the marketing department during my last few years, I focused heavily on patient referrals. The referrals came from various sources—privately or through our network of medical groups, insurance companies, religious groups, private organizations, and other medical facilities.

On difficult or complex referrals, I would request Dr. Luck's assistance for direction and resolution—those cases that required special considerations medically or involved other issues or ramifications. We worked together on countless situations and on extremely difficult and complex cases. The following are two examples that show how Dr. Luck took that extra step to help me fulfill requests—extra steps which I personally appreciated because of the end result.

I received a telephone call from a woman in New York City around seven o'clock one morning. Her son was attending summer classes at the USC campus located a few blocks from our hospital. He apparently was having a severe neck problem and needed to see a doctor. The mother was really concerned and she had been upset trying to address the situation. I mentioned that it was only seven in the morning in California, but we needed to put a plan in place. She had insurance coverage for her son and I requested that she fax me copies of the card and other pertinent information. I asked for her son's telephone number and informed her that I would take care of everything and get back to her. I called the son to bring him up to date and to tell him to stand by for my return call regarding his doctor's appointment. The mother sounded so concerned and distraught that it was a priority for me to have him seen by one of our physicians that day. Arranging spur-of-the-moment physician appointments could be difficult, as offices had full schedules on their patient days. However, the mother was so anguished I wanted to get her son's needs expeditiously addressed.

That particular morning, I called every office and no doctor was available to work this patient into his schedule. I knew that Dr. Luck had a very tight schedule that day in his personal office, and, between patients, I stopped by to tell him my dilemma. When he learned that I needed to fulfill my promise to the patient's mother, he said he would see the patient during his lunch hour. After examining the patient the doctor recommended that the student stop his classes at USC and return to New York and immediately start physical therapy and other follow-up care.

The son was a nice young man and eager to follow Dr. Luck's instructions. The worried mother was grateful—she even mailed me a nice thank you letter and a check for a dinner and a social evening. I turned the check over to our children's foundation and thanked her for her kindness. That young man's concerned mother was so on edge when she called me so early in the morning, I simply could not have postponed an appointment for another day unless it had been absolutely imperative. Dr. Luck and I both realized her concerns and, as usual, he bailed me out to fulfill the need. She was so appreciative and had no need to send a check expressing her gratitude—but she did. It was a nice gift that we graciously accepted as a donation for one of our children's charity programs.

Another mother called me one day from back East regarding her daughter who was about nineteen years old and who had had multiple surgeries on her knee and the lower part of her leg.

A friend had mentioned to the mother that our hospital had provided excellent care to one of her family members and suggested she call us for help. She informed me that her daughter was actually working in her surgeon's office and her condition was such that she was between crutches and a wheel chair. I asked that she send copies of her daughter's medical history, which turned out to be voluminous, and I asked Dr. Luck to review it. I wasn't certain what Dr. Luck would suggest, but I knew he would review the medical records and come up with something, even if it meant having the woman come to our hospital. Fortunately, within one hundred miles from the mother's home there was a colleague of Dr. Luck, and he referred the patient to him.

This took place during the summer months and the patient had hoped to start college in the fall. She wanted to become a doctor, but was very distraught and discouraged about her orthopaedic condition. I instructed the mother to be certain she mention to the doctor that Dr. Luck had referred her daughter to him. The patient saw the doctor—he cancelled his vacation in order to perform surgery on her and monitor her continued care until school started. After surgery the patient threw away her crutches and discarded her wheel chair—one happy mother and daughter.

The mother sent a letter of appreciation to Dr. Luck and me with pictures of her beautiful daughter standing very tall. Needless to say, Dr. Luck and I were very happy just taking that extra step to help someone so many miles away.

It was also good to remember that another grateful parent had referred the mother to Orthopaedic Hospital. Good deeds and consistency brought forth a chain reaction that was gratifying to all concerned.

My colleague, Chuck, the administrative director of the Joint Replacement Institute (JRI) at Orthopaedic Hospital, informed me that a young Canadian physician in his late twenties had temporarily joined their medical staff. He said that he was French Canadian and had been practicing medicine in Ottawa, but hailed from Quebec City. He said, "When you get a chance, just stop by and meet a fellow Canadian. You will really like him." Shortly thereafter, I went to his office and, before introducing myself, I started to sing, "O Canada." He laughed and we introduced ourselves—he was Paul Beaulé, M.D.

Chuck was right. I do not recall ever meeting anyone for the first time that I liked so immediately. My first impression has been lasting, and, since that time, I have never faltered from my original observation of him.

He was to spend one year at the JRI and, upon completion, spend several months at Good Samaritan Hospital, my former employer. While there, he would be under the tutelage of another physician for an additional orthopaedic specialty. At the end of his first three months, I informed Chuck that Dr. Beaulé had blended into our little group so easily. I was really happy he was onboard with us. Chuck concurred and we three really bonded so well, sharing the same work standards, moral outlook, and—befittingly—crazy sense of humor.

At the end of six months, I met with Chuck and said that our doctor's assignment at our hospital was almost half over. By that time, he had become very important to us—an integral part of our vocational/professional lives. I soon realized he would be going to Good Samaritan Hospital and he would continue to see us, but, beyond that, he would be returning to Canada. I did not want to face that eventuality, though it kept cropping up like a noose around my neck. I had grown so fond of him, as he and Chuck and I had become a happy troika.

After many years away from The Hospital of the Good Samaritan, I found that one of the good friends I'd had while working there was now managing the business office. I called her when Dr. Beaulé was ready to join their staff for several months to arrange with her to have lunch with the doctor and me.

Over the years, we had remained friends and I informed her privately that this young man was super special to me—a kindred spirit. I wanted her to be certain he was well taken care of during his stay there. We three had a nice lunch and it worked out well for him. While at Good Samaritan Hospital he did keep in touch with us. However, I kept worrying about having to face his day of departure and his return to Canada. He had a wonderful wife, who was also a medical professional, practicing in dentistry. They had three beautiful children—two daughters and one son.

One day before completing his assignment at Good Samaritan Hospital, Dr. Beaulé stopped by my office and immediately closed my door. He sat down, broadly smiling, and said that he and his wife had decided they wanted to remain in California. Further, he stated that he wanted to return to Orthopaedic Hospital and establish his medical practice in the Joint Replacement Unit. I was shocked, but overwhelmed, as nothing could have pleased me more. He asked if I could help him get established in his practice, and I said with elation, "Absolutely! I will do anything I can to keep you here."

I never thought twice about committing myself to helping him build a solid foundation for his medical practice. Additionally, he had all of the basic ingredients: he was a great physician and surgeon, an honorable and moral young man, and totally dedicated to his wonderful wife and family, which I most admired. I was so proud of the way he conducted himself with everyone. Several of our physicians, due to my transparency, surmised how important he was to me. They went out of their way to tell me laudatory comments about his professional skills and conduct—none of which surprised me.

Through Chuck and his group, we got the paperwork started to cover all of the ramifications of treatment and third-party payer sign-up requirements for new physicians. The process included applications for sign-up with the various intermediaries and insurance companies, medical groups, etc. He already had an excellent rapport with the medical staff and he had assisted many of the doctors on their difficult cases. He was also extremely accommodating to his patients, spending sufficient time with them until recovery. He treated his patients and hospital staff alike in a courteous and very friendly manner.

I was developing a good rapport working with one of our newer medical groups and I was trying to increase our referral base with them. The facilitating manager and I worked very well together. He had a personal friend who was in his late twenties or early thirties who had had two prior hip surgeries and his surgeon was calling for a third one. The patient, incidentally, was also employed in the healthcare field. The patient had become somewhat disgruntled and wanted a second opinion before he proceeded to approve a third surgery. In working with the medical group manager, I suggested that the patient come to our hospital and to have Dr. Beaulé examine him. The patient had continuously been on crutches and was really discouraged with the entire medical process. The final result was that he had a third surgery with Dr. Beaulé, and the patient threw away his crutches and he is extremely grateful to have a total recovery. That patient is in the vanguard of this doctor's greatest fans, along with the facilitating manager and their entire medical group. They love him.

I had been working successfully with a medical group in Tahiti for a few years. Tahiti is a popular tourist haven, particularly for those on cruise ships and others on direct package flights. Unfortunately, injuries do occur for vacationers—often related to hiking or surfing accidents. Also, orthopaedic problems occur, particularly to the elderly tourists.

American tourists who are injured in Tahiti and who require medical services are sent via air service to California because it is the closest point from Tahiti. Our hospital became the hospital of choice for most of the orthopaedic patients. I believe initially the group of physicians we work with in Tahiti learned about us through the Internet. Their first request for a medical transfer was referred to me. I initiated the transfer of that patient and remained the key person in facilitating all transfers thereafter. Air France was very accommodating in transferring these patients who required individual gurney services.

When Dr. Beaulé joined our staff, the French doctors in Tahiti found him a windfall, as he spoke French fluently. They were tremendously agog at being able to have him as a key physician in the loop. It also enabled them to send their notes and reports in both French and English. Dr. Beaulé took care of several of their cases and it was a beneficial exchange. They were so happy that he was onboard. To assist the Tahitian doctors, he was available to help in the further referral of any cases referred to us, if other services were to be provided elsewhere.

Dr. Beaulé's involvement assured all concerned that nothing got lost in the translation. They appreciated his availability in the screening process and the decision-making process as this medical group was so many miles away. The French doctors in Tahiti very quickly perceived Dr. Beaulé's adroitness in dispatching his requests and recommendations, and for the transfer and care of their patients at our hospital. And they followed Dr. Beaulé's instructions precisely.

One of the large medical groups that sent patients to us routinely had one medical facility in the desert that never used our hospital. It was actually a bone of contention with me as to why they had no occasion to use our services. It seemed that the orthopaedic coverage in their region was able to accommodate their cases. It was somewhat of an anomaly, as we received countless referrals from their other medical groups. However, one of the physicians in the medical group contacted me to see if one of our physicians would accept an extremely difficult orthopaedic case—loaded with other complications. I requested the physician send me copies of their reports so that we could have the case reviewed. I spoke with Dr. Beaulé and, upon reading the reports, he agreed without hesitancy to see the patient.

Prior to his initial visit with our doctor, the patient called and said that no one in the desert would touch his complicated case, and he wanted to afford our doctor the opportunity to bow out. Dr. Beaulé still firmly agreed to see the patient. He performed the surgery and all went well. I recall casually asking him a few days after the surgery about this patient, and identified it as a very difficult case. He simply replied, "Everything went fine!"

I have felt a very personal and special bond with this young doctor. It is also gratifying to see what an accomplished physician he became, as demonstrated by the accolades he has received from his patients, peers, and associates. Modesty is deeply ingrained into his being.

Working with him has been a very fulfilling experience, as I am so proud of what he has achieved. We maintained high standards but had fun, too. In being with him came a renewal of my fond memories of that wonderful French Canadian family that was so endearing to our family during my many difficult childhood years when I was motherless during the horrible Depression.

Dr. Beaulé has since returned to Canada after accepting an excellent position at a teaching center. I believe the university is very fortunate to have this wonderful physician and surgeon on staff. I am certain that the union will be mutually beneficial to the university and Dr. Beaulé. He is most proud of his French Canadian background and a very proud Canadian (or *Canadien*!).

My years at Orthopaedic Hospital were fulfilling, and I enjoyed working with my colleagues tremendously. It was a great hospital and I stayed longer than I had anticipated, as it was a worthy experience and a great place to throw in the towel to complete my career. I do keep in touch with Dr. Luck, who stated on one of my recent visits, "Gus, you will always be a part of Orthopaedic Hospital."

Summation

When I was very young, my father told me the following story that left a profound impact on me. He personally stressed the importance of presenting one's self in a favorable light and respecting the needs of others. Throughout my childhood and youth, my father would tell anecdotes that carried specific messages. Thus, we would have the engagement of the story and, simultaneously, gather the message. I believe the reader will note that I also make a similar delivery.

Here is the story: Art was a great family friend who was married and had a devoted wife and three daughters, all younger than members of our family. Art was, by vocation, a machinist and apparently an excellent machine tool maker. However, during the bleak Depression years he had great difficulty in securing any type of employment. In stature he was very tall, slim, and always extremely well dressed, even in casual or work-type clothing. Toward the end of the Depression, Art applied to see if there were any open positions at a bed and mattress factory. He approached a young man as he entered the office. The young man, without any inquiry, said somewhat caustically, "We have no job openings." Art tried to pursue the conversation with him. The young man kept saying, "We have nothing to offer!" By innuendo, he attempted to give Art the bum's rush. Suddenly, the owner appeared and Art calmly, but mendaciously, informed him that he represented a large logging company. His mission was to order two hundred beds for the logger's sleeping quarters. Art said, "In view of the reception I received from your employee, I shall go elsewhere to place an order to someone more appreciative and deserving of our business." Immediately, the owner apologized profusely for the bad conduct of his employee—but to no avail. Art slowly walked down the street in anticipation. Suddenly, the young man came running toward him apologizing and begging him to place the order as he had just been fired over the incident. Art said, "You should be fired and replaced with a more deserving person."

This story is an interesting example of human behavior that addresses several salient points:

• It took place during the horrible Depression era of massive unemployment.

239

- The young man should have realized it was a privilege that he had a full-time position. Along with others, thousands of his contemporaries were out of work. Instead of realizing his good fortune, he demeaned others such as our friend.

- Regardless of the circumstances, the young employee should have presented himself as a responsible and respectful employee on behalf of his employer and organization. The onus was with him, as an employee, to conduct himself in an appropriate manner.

- The young man's assumption that our family friend was seeking employment was correct; however, he could not have known that for certain, and he should not have applied a double standard.

- Good business acumen would have been applied if the young man treated each person consistently equally.

- The curt employee should have offered our friend an opportunity to pursue the conversation further. Had Art mentioned that he was applying for a job, the employee should have informed him politely that there were no open positions. He should have demonstratively shown some compassion. If Art wished to pursue the conversation further, the employee should have afforded him the opportunity to speak directly with the employer. It would have involved only an additional step or two to change the entire situation.

- The employer acted in good faith. Regardless of the circumstances, bad news travels fast. Our family friend could have passed his negative experience to others and they could have passed it to others, creating a wide-spread negative image for that company.

- However, the employer practiced good judgment and equitability.

- This organization at the time was probably pleading for more business. The young employee, if he remained a loose cannon, could have created other detrimental situations that could cause loss to the employer.

My family friend's action certainly took all of the above thoughts quickly into consideration. His intervention was beneficial to the employer and, hopefully, to the employee as well, providing him with a lesson to be learned. When the Depression ended, our friend became a successful self-employed toolmaker with purchasing power.

My niece Michele attended a magnet school in Woodland Hills several years ago. The school was very progressive, and students were coming from all parts of greater Los Angeles, commuting by school bus daily. One of her classes was a course in typing, and her teacher afforded family members in the business community or others to be guest speakers. The purpose was to enlighten the students by broadening their exposure to the business world. My niece asked if I would be interested in coming to her class to conduct a session. I accepted and thought it was a great opportunity to see her in a classroom setting and to meet her fellow students. And I had been interested in the concept of magnet schools, which offer specialized courses that draw students from a wide urban region, with a partial aim at desegregation.

At the time, I was at St. John's Regional Medical Center, and I decided to take admission materials to class and have the students admit Mickey Mouse to our hospital. For sample forms, I completed in advance the required documentation, stating that the patient lived at Walt Disney Studios and was married to Minnie Mouse, etc.

The teacher was delighted with my approach. The students diligently typed their admission information on the blank sample forms that I had provided. They seemed to be having a great time in the process. I attempted to authenticate this exercise as being in a work-related environment. I believe that I was successful. Their enthusiasm was refreshing and contagious, and I enjoyed being with them. I quickly noticed they were all very attentive and well-mannered youngsters, and they loved the concept of admitting Mickey Mouse to our hospital.

While they were busily typing the documents, I casually mentioned to the teacher that I believed one of the most important skills I had acquired was the ability to type proficiently. When she heard this comment, she immediately instructed her students to stop and listen. Said she, "I want Mr. Munro to repeat to you just what he has said to me—his comments are extremely important, especially coming from a successful administrative healthcare professional."

On a personal note, my niece seemed slightly blasé when I first arrived, and she greeted me at the front entrance with one of her class companions. However, before conducting the class, her teacher and I had coffee in their break room. At that time, she informed me that Michele had been very excited and had been overzealously anticipating my arrival to their classroom. I found her comments timely and apropos. It was a very enjoyable day for me. The teacher assigned a special task for the students to perform at their following typing class. The class was instructed by their teacher to compose and type a thank you letter to me for being a guest speaker. As youngsters in the eighth grade, they did extremely well and I was very impressed. It had been a very pleasant, rewarding, and fulfilling experience for me.

While teaching these youngsters, the thought did occur to me that, at near their age, I was bowing out of school as a dropout. As a mature adult, I found it hard to believe that I had, at such a young age, thrown in the towel so to speak. It would have been absolutely inconceivable to me, to see my niece falter and, at about the same age, drop out of school. It would have been unrealistic, unthinkable, and unimaginative for that to happen to her. But it had happened to me.

When I dropped out I had no idea of the consequences I would suffer, but my decision haunted me in the years that followed.

Teaching this typing class was profoundly rewarding to me:

- This was my first experience in actually teaching a class in a schoolroom setting. All of my teaching experience had been work-related and always in an adult setting.

- On my road to recovery from having been a dropout, typing had been my initial step in getting my plan in motion following the inspiring Dutch uncle speech I received from George, the University of British Columbia theological student who inspired me to get myself going in the right direction.

- In actuality, in terms of a career, typing had been my most treasured skill. Throughout the years in the petroleum industry, executives working on a Saturday, without a secretary or typing ability, would ask for my assistance to type an important letter or memorandum for them—the requests were always humorous … "Help me!"

- In the beginning of the computer era, many of my colleagues had no typing skills; they were forced to learn the basics to prepare their own memoranda, letters, and reports. Internal retrenchment lessened our secretarial services.

- I typed my father's business letters for him and he was quite impressed. Complimentary recognition from my father was normally very infrequent. On one occasion, I prepared an important letter for him. He was almost speechless when he read it. He later commented that it had been incredibly well written.

- Also, to gain more experience, I prepared business letters for others. The process was a two-fold exercise—I improved my basic typing and honed my letter-writing skills.

- I started to learn my communication skills when I worked at the CPR Tele-graph Office. Brevity was extremely important, as the senders of cables, tele-grams, and night letters were charged based on the actual word count.

As I mentioned earlier, I was very successful in conducting classes in Alaska for our nursing personnel. Throughout my career in healthcare, I conducted many classes for my departmental personnel on various subjects—all work-related. I have made numerous presentations to groups promotionally presenting the vari-ous services offered in whichever facility I was working for at the time. I have made countless presentations in hospital settings and throughout the community on various topics, including the Medicare and Medicaid programs, Workers' Compensation, and other third-party payers, intermediaries, etc. Presentations for me were basic and commonplace; however, I never forgot that I was repre-senting both my hospital and my department—I always exercised decorum.

I tried to make my presentations interesting and I did insert humor into those sessions and tried to evoke audience participation. I demonstrated compassion, politeness, and patience, particularly addressing complicated Medicare issues to our elderly members in the audience. Senior groups were most important to our hospitals and represented a substantial number of our patients. Addressing their needs was of paramount importance.

It seems an ambiguity that I have felt so comfortable in a classroom setting, having left school in my primary years. My workplace along with whatever edu-cational programs I pursued—my entire environment—became a classroom set-ting for me. In other words, I learned on the job—empirically and by osmosis. This may sound pompous and egotistical, but, candidly, I met very few persons in the work scene who truly impressed me by their intellect or adeptness. Further, in many cases, their individual general performance in discharging assigned responsibilities didn't impress me either. And that assessment is based on work-ing closely with upper-level management throughout the years in both Canada and the United States.

Apart from the parties and poker games, my father did provide me with great input that followed me and provided positive influence throughout my life. He instilled the good qualities that I have possessed in showing compassion to the employees who have reported to me in addressing their work problems and indi-vidual needs. He always stated simplistically, "Do the right thing!" While I was still working in the sawmill, he was an outside foreman over a group of men, and he discussed labor relations issues with me. Paradoxically, he was extremely lib-eral but very dedicated to the wellbeing of his company and his superintendent.

Dad was very cognizant of his role as intermediary when occasions arose such as mandatory reduction in the workforce during quiet periods. He worked hard to juggle and placate to keep everyone happy. He was exemplary in reducing his own hours in deference to those with larger families to support. In those days, he worked from his head and with his heart, and not a procedural manual, to ensure equitability.

Over the years I have received many accolades presented in the form of speeches, plaques, statuary, and framed written documents, all relating to my favorable relationships and my work ethic, both within organizations and in the community. Years ago, my father gave me the motto, "Treat others as you wish to be treated yourself." It is that simple, and I know many well-educated persons who have devoted hours taking programs to try and improve their relationships with people, and they still falter in trying to achieve that goal. Many simply just don't get it. To treat people equitably, one must respect their privacy and confidentiality and sagaciously, but quietly, analyze their point of view in addressing difficult or controversial situations.

I have experienced many circumstances as a director in having to pacify disgruntled patients and/or their family members due to poor manners exhibited on the part of one of my employees or managers. In these types of situations, one must seek compromise and resolution instead of being bellicose and screaming in the trenches. Taking the high road in an amicable way is most rewarding to all concerned; just being right does not always garner compromise, resolution, and goodwill.

In any managerial or directorship position I have held, realizing my strengths and weaknesses, I meticulously tried to develop my work plan to be commensurate with what I had to offer. In the process, I carefully observed the people who reported to me regarding their strengths and weaknesses and how we could all unite as a viable and forceful team. In that process there can be some give and take. My personal druthers favor a management team such as the ones I myself have fostered—strictly bread-and-butter, and working in the trenches with total involvement.

I have been perplexed throughout the years when looking at my unorthodox limited educational background and measuring it against my vocational history. I am somewhat surprised that I unequivocally never ever sensed that I was in over my head. Strangely enough, I found myself far more able to accept the challenges of the position—more so than many of my predecessors. I would review their departmental manuals and other instructional material (or notice the lack of

them) and recognize the need to rewrite and restructure many of their procedures.

I also had the liberty and accessibility to assume more responsibilities, such as
marketing and other promotional activities. I seemed to be in the vanguard of
those initiating and developing new programs. In California and Alaska I found
myself working as a maverick and advocate on certain intermediary issues relating
to the Medi-cal and Medicaid programs based on the hospital's perspective,
addressing those issues that were not always clearly defined. This also applied to
quick-fix changes to accommodate the other side with no benefit to the healthcare facility. Being in the forefront, we had to work in tandem, which was challenging for all.

I received excellent annual employee reviews from every employer. The only
request of most of my employers was that I try and reduce my hours, which fell
on deaf ears. Unfortunately, it was one balance I never seemed to personally
achieve. I left every position in good stead and I am certain I could have been
reinstated if I cared to return. Four of my former employers requested my return;
and I had to gratefully decline. I have been a complete, supportive, and loyal an
employee to every organization listed on my resume.

In the overall picture, I have been truly blessed with working with some of the
most wonderful people I have ever known. Many still remain my friends today,
while others I have lost touch with, and, of course, many have departed. I am so
grateful to George, the University of British Columbia student who told me to
get my ass moving in the right direction. If you listen, you may find that another
person can change your direction in life. During my exchange of dialogue with
George, as he delivered his Dutch uncle speech, he related his comments to my
circumstances, rather than my overall potential. This had a profound impact on
me that made me pause and ponder.

For some strange reason, I accepted what he said as worth considering and I
immediately put a plan in place. Up to that point, aside from being a grade-
school dropout, I had been a child goat herder, chief cook and bottle washer, busboy, farmhand, popcorn maker, and sawmill conveyor robot. With that limited
vocational background, what the hell did I know?

I simply took one day at a time without a master plan. I tried to improve vocationally and enhance my educational background in the process. At that time,
unbeknownst to myself, I was an empiricist—a student of observation—and a
pragmatist. I did not have a winding road to travel. My road was very clear and

straight-ahead. I started at the T. Eaton Company in their stockroom, and I realized I had no where to go but up—as soon as I put the wheels in motion.

- I learned that I was quickly recognized for having good work habits and the ability to grasp my individual responsibilities and fulfill my duties proficiently. Thus, the onus to be productive and participatory was with me.

- The recognition was hardest to accept. Good work habits were instilled in my being. I was unaccustomed to receive such laudatory, ongoing praise.

- I had been blessed with good manners. I worked well with all members of our staff and, importantly, with our customers—always taking that extra step.

- Being chief cook and bottle washer had provided me with self-motivation.

- Humility was my middle name. The constant kudos given to me in the workplace, I found extremely hard to accept. I felt like a fraud. If they only knew …

- While I realized that, with my very limited background, my options for any future advancement could be very limited, I simply took one day at a time.

- Taking classes in typing and bookkeeping brought my confidence level up. My octopus-type behavior afforded me an opportunity to fulfill multiple assignments in any department where I worked.

- Working at the CPR Telegraph Office was immediately challenging in improving my typing skills, spelling, and vocabulary. I also learned to communicate proficiently with business personnel from all levels, along with the general public.

- Being a supervisor in my early twenties—with a staffing complement aged up to sixty-five—was, surprisingly, a piece of cake. I never had a moment's concern. With teamwork and respect for others, we worked together to get the job done.

- At British American Oil, I was under the mentorship of Jack. Through emulation and osmosis, I developed good communication skills, both written and oral. Frankly, I had had a good basic grounding at the CPR—writing clearly and concisely. I quietly listened, observed, and emulated.

- I developed my basic marketing skills interacting with our agents and sales representatives, along with our customers—putting all of the pieces together.

- While at British American Oil, I was informed on several occasions that I had been the most promoted person in the shortest period of time—in their entire western office. This was totally bewildering for this dropout to comprehend.

- When starting Standard Oil, I had a good work background; however, scholastically, all I had was a blank piece of paper. My solace was in keeping this my hidden secret.

- Ironically, aside from just learning the Los Angeles and Southern California landscape, everything else quickly fell into place. Work-wise, my time spent at Standard Oil was refining general procedures, training, and helping my many colleagues, who all had that completed "piece of paper." At the time, I self-imposingly thought it was a demeaning atmosphere; however, looking back, it was a very constructive environment—surprisingly so. I really grew.

- In hindsight, I never understood if my "blank piece of paper" was in actuality my "Waterloo" or a blessing in disguise, providing me with fortitude to forge ahead. I had little time for philosophical thinking. My daily plate was crammed full of mundane, bread-and-butter issues.

- Richfield Oil became the apex of my career in the petroleum industry. (Except for Jack's frightening "AR joy rides"—I still shudder at the thought of them.) Ironically, Jack was my biggest fan ever, showering me with accolades galore. They had me scheduled for the corporate office—another rung or two up the ladder. I bowed out, but left with a feeling of total gratitude for the success and recognition I received. It was a wonderful time and place. And the infamous Harry Swisher turned out to be my guardian angel—a decent man.

- The Hospital of the Good Samaritan in 1964 was one of the top five hospitals in the country. In terms of on-the-job-training, my position there was my Harvard—vocational finishing school. With the title of consultant, I was given free range to get involved in everything but direct patient care. My colleague at Richfield Oil had been right when he suggested I try hospital administration. It was a perfect fit.

- At St. John's Regional Medical Center, I was able to accept more specific responsibilities, applying the wonderful training and experience that I had acquired at Good Samaritan. It became my home and it was a family setting. In terms of favorites, it hit the top of my list. I was extremely proud of my contributions to that hospital and my involvement with their medical staff and our community at large. The sisters were marvelous!

- Providence in Anchorage was the most challenging position to me. I worked very long and hard hours to develop and maintain a good standard within my departments. However, I loved the hospital, the setting, and the wonderful people of Alaska. I broadened my background in working with all governmental services and agencies, and welcomed my involvement with the various media—print, radio and television. It was very exciting—I was filled with sort of a pioneering spirit in that vast beautiful wilderness. It was a great adventure for me.

- Delano Regional Medical Center was a brief twenty-month excursion, but was a pleasant and rewarding experience. I wanted to experience working at a hospital in a smaller community. I gained valuable knowledge in that setting. And maintained a high accountability level.

- Orthopaedic Hospital was the end of my long vocational journey. As I started working there at age sixty-one, I thought my tenure would be about four years. The timing and circumstances were such that I remained there for eleven years. Actually, I would have remained longer if it had not been for the negative effect on my annuities. Prolonging retirement would have increased taxation implications.

- Orthopaedic Hospital and I fit together like a hand in a glove. My many years in healthcare were evident in the way I conducted my duties. I always developed and maintained excellent working relationships with physicians, and Orthopaedic Hospital was home to my favorite medical group. Most of our physicians had their offices within our hospital campus, which afforded me the ability to build lasting relationships with them and their office personnel. We were so participatory—physicians and their office staff alike—we were really an extended family. When I had any special concerns, I would select the physician most appropriate to address the subject. I felt a very personal involvement with the entire hospital and total medical complex. It was a great setting in which to complete my working years.

Whatever path we take, whatever responsibilities are given to us, we must consider personal accountability: What are our personal expectations? What do others believe our role is in terms of fulfilling their needs, whether they are of a personal nature or work-related?

Success is an individual assessment. And success can be achieved through any work endeavor or environment. Whatever is the task, we are there to perform to the best of our ability and to work with others affording them our consideration and respect. In the process, we can hope to receive the same considerations from them. The fulfillment of a job well done truly comes from within and not from others. Yes, we love hearing laudatory recognition and support for a job well done, but I believe that self-gratification ranks a notch higher!

A special closing thought: My father was the love of my life. When he passed away, I continually dreamed of him for about seven years and would wake up in the middle of night wondering if he was in my presence. I hope that he would be pleased and proud of my accomplishments. I am thankful to him for giving me such basic grounding in both work-related endeavors and in addressing the needs of others. I simply picked up the pieces and gave it my best. His goodness is within me and unequivocally supersedes the title of this book, *A Full House—But Empty!*

978-0-595-43719-1
0-595-43719-2

Printed in the United States
94895LV00004B/64-72/A